UNSPOKEN
Desires

UNSPOKEN
Desires

Real People Talk About Sexual
Experiences and Fantasies They
Hide from Their Partners

Iris and Steven Finz

St. Martin's Press
New York

Design by Heidi A.S. Eriksen

ISBN 0-312-25344-3

This book is dedicated to
all those who helped us
better understand ourselves and
each other by sharing with us and
our readers their unspoken desires.

CONTENTS

Introduction

This is a book about the sexual thoughts and desires that relationship-partners keep secret from each other. When we were gathering material for it, one of the women we interviewed told us that her husband always makes love to her slowly, thoroughly, and considerately. Then she added, wistfully, that she sometimes wishes she had an additional husband who would occasionally throw her down on the floor or across the dining room table and use her unceremoniously for his own satisfaction.

We were tempted to suggest that she tell her husband about this wish and ask if he was interested in helping her fulfill it, but that was not our job. We conduct many interviews and discuss sex with many people, but never as therapists, or sociologists, or any other kind of ologists. We just listen attentively and report on what we've heard. We may draw a few conclusions and we may incorporate some of them into our writing. For the most part, though, we hope that our readers, each in his or her own way, will find their own lessons among the experiences we describe.

The woman's wish for an additional husband typifies the phenomenon that furnishes the theme for this book. Most people harbor secret erotic wishes that they are unwilling to discuss with their mates. The reasons for this reticence may be quite complicated.

Monogamy is our society's norm. That means that each of us is expected to find satisfaction with a single sex partner. However, no two people are identical. Sexuality varies from one person to another the way fingerprints do. A wife may have a sexual need that she believes to be incompatible with her husband's personality. A husband may harbor an erotic desire that he thinks will be offensive to his wife. So they stifle the urge to discuss these needs, burying them deep within the secret vaults of private consciousness.

This may cause the unspoken desire to take on an exaggerated importance. It may become an obsession, its repression a source of disappointment and chronic dissatisfaction. During sex, each partner may focus on his or her secret need, to the exclusion of everything else, until the union between them becomes a collection of separate erotic experiences that both are having at the same time and place, but neither is sharing with the other.

Almost all the people with whom we spoke admitted keeping erotic secrets from their mates. Some of them said that we were the first persons they ever told about these hidden urges. Most felt guilty about concealing their true thoughts from their partners. Many were ashamed about the desires themselves, believing that their private fantasies marked them as weird or perverted.

Readers of our previous books have told us that they were relieved to learn that their sexual activities were not as unusual as they had believed them to be. Until our books were published, these people had no way of really knowing what their neighbors and contemporaries were doing behind closed bedroom doors. As a result, they had formed disturbing ideas about what was "normal" or "unnatural." It was only by exposure to the sexuality of others that they were able to recognize the trends that made them a part of the human race, rather than set them apart from it.

We hope that the stories in this book will help our readers to realize that they are not alone in keeping erotic secrets. In fact, there's a good chance that their spouses and partners also have a few. That knowledge may be enough to make most people more comfortable with their own sexuality. In addition, readers of this book are likely to discover that there are others who share their personal unspoken desires. They are not so weird or perverted, after all.

We do not believe it is possible to find a random sampling of people who are willing to speak honestly about their sex lives. So we have never attempted to take a survey or to determine what percentage of the population likes a particular kind of sex. The stories we have heard range widely, covering every possible branch of the erotic imagination. Some are so unusual that little would be accomplished by repeating them. There are themes, though, that seem to recur with great frequency. The stories we have chosen help to establish these themes, each of which is represented by a separate chapter. It is our hope and belief that among them you will find one that reminds you of yourself.

UNSPOKEN
Desires

ONE

Take Me Now!

*I*n the Victorian age, women were not supposed to enjoy sex. They had an obligation to their husbands and were required to feel some emotional satisfaction in fulfilling it, but were prohibited from deriving any physical pleasure from doing so. When giving vent to his animal nature, a true gentleman finished the nasty act as quickly as possible so that he would not subject his mate to excessive stress or temptation.

Now, a hundred or so years later, we have come to recognize that women have the same sexual needs and the same sexual rights as men and are entitled to all the physical pleasure they can legitimately derive. The true gentleman is sensitive to the desires of women and adept in the erotic arts. He educates himself about the female body so that he can help his mate to achieve satisfaction.

Sometimes, however, this change in expectations makes demands that contemporary men and women find hard to fulfill. Foreplay takes energy, but life in modern society may exhaust all the strength a person has, whether male or female. As a result, many people long, at least occasionally, for sex that is quick and unceremonious. They may suppress that yearning, though, and keep it secret, because they believe it is not consistent with the philosophy of our times.

The stories in this chapter suggest the irony that may result. Herman fondly remembers early sexual encounters, clumsy but exciting, that were fit into stolen moments, but is ashamed to confess to his wife that he desires to re-experience this kind of sex. Mary wishes she could be taken swiftly and without preamble, but is unable to admit this to either of her patient and considerate lovers.

Wouldn't it be nice if Herman learned that his wife wanted the same thing that Mary wants? Wouldn't Mary's life improve if either of her lovers turned out to need the same kind of sex that Herman needs? Nothing like this will happen, however, as long as the hunger that they experience remains an unspoken desire.

Down and Dirty

*H*erman, thirty-two, is a firefighter. He says that advances in fire prevention have reduced the number of fires to be fought, so he has plenty of time to work on developing his body. Perhaps this accounts for his muscular physique. He is six feet one inch tall and weighs in the vicinity of two-hundred pounds, all of it solid and none of it superfluous. His light brown hair is close-cropped. His eyes are a darker shade of brown.

Norma and I have been married for, what, almost six years now. We've got a pretty good life. All in all, I'd say that our sex is pretty satisfying. Maybe more so for her than for me.

Like that old song says, Norma likes a lover with a slow hand. To her, sex is nothing without a long, drawn-out buildup. Lots of foreplay. Lots of whispering, kissing, touching. Pleasing her sexually takes an awful lot of work. But I pride myself on taking care of her needs, and I don't think she is ever unsatisfied after one of our lovemaking sessions.

To tell you the truth, though, I don't think we make love as often as we could, because her preference is not always my preference. Lots of times, I feel that if I had my way, I'd like it just plain down and dirty. You know: jump on, ram it in, pop my nuts, and jump off. Hell, I'd still be gentle, but I'd just like to do it without all that tenderness that she's expecting.

I've never said anything to her about it, because I just

know she wouldn't understand. I've even heard her say that men who disregard their wife's needs are no better than animals. I wouldn't want her to lose respect for me, so that's a part of me that I keep hidden from her.

Maybe it all started with my first sex experience. I'll never forget it. I was about sixteen and there was a girl in the neighborhood a couple of years older than me who used to fuck for money. My friends decided it was time for me to lose my virginity and so they set me up with her. They all chipped in to pay her. It couldn't have cost very much, though, because it didn't take but a few minutes.

I met her on the roof of the apartment building she lived in. There was nobody else around at the moment, but you never knew when someone would show up. So, right from the start, there was a sense of urgency about it. I wanted to look at her and feel her titties, but she said there was no time for that. As soon as we got onto the roof, she pulled up her skirt. She had nothing on underneath it.

I just got the barest glimpse of her pussy before she had my pants down around my ankles and my dick in her hand. While I was still in a daze, she had worked it into her and was humping back and forth for all she was worth. After just a few seconds, I felt myself getting ready to come. I wanted to put it off, to stall and make the sensation last as long as possible. But she dug her fingers into my ass and kept humping until I just couldn't hold out any longer.

When I went off, it was like a cannon. As soon as I was done, she stepped back away from me, lowered her skirt, and headed for the stairway. By the time I got my pants back in place, she was gone.

Looking back on it, you might think that it was too fast and cold to be really exciting. That wasn't the way it affected me, though. I had been jerking off every day ever since I figured out how—sometimes a few times a day. This was my first experience with a real live woman. To me, it was the most exciting thing that ever could have happened. After that, I thought about it all the time, especially when I was masturbating in my room at the end of a day.

I really didn't have any other sexual contact with women until I was about eighteen and I started dating. I saw a few girls, mostly the sisters of my friends, but nothing much ever happened. Like a lot of people my age, I was kind of awkward about sex and just never made the right moves.

By the time I was nineteen, I had passed the tests and was enrolled in the firefighter's academy. A woman named Amy was there, too, training for a career in firefighting just like the rest of us. She was the only female in the academy and so she received a lot of male attention. It looked to me like she was working her way through all the guys in the class. This gave me the courage I needed to ask her out. She said yes right away, and I took her to a movie.

I don't remember the picture, because the whole time we sat there, I was trying to figure out a way of getting into her pants. After the movie, I asked if she'd like to get something to eat, but she suggested going back to her apartment. She said her parents were out for the evening and we could be alone there. The sound of that excited me. Maybe tonight would be my night. Maybe I'd score. Boy, I certainly wasn't expecting what happened next.

Her place was only a few blocks from the movie theater, and we walked at a pretty good clip. She led me up two flights of stairs and then unlocked the apartment door. As soon as I stepped in behind her, she closed the door and locked it. "I want you to fuck me," she said. "Right here and right now."

I was startled. By the time I regained any semblance of composure, she had stripped off her pants and panties and was stretched out on her back on the floor with her legs spread and her feet pointed at the ceiling. "Come on," she said. "Don't waste any time. I want your cock and I want it right away. Quick, before my parents get home."

I couldn't believe my good fortune, but I had enough sense

not to stand there analyzing it. Instead, I started tearing my clothes off. After my pants and shorts, I began working on my shirt. She practically shouted, "Never mind that. Fuck me, now!"

So I did. I jumped on top of her and started bucking around until my cock found its way into her. I still don't know how I managed it. The second I entered her, she started moaning, real loud. Next thing I knew, I was coming. And coming. And coming.

All the sexual energy that had been mounting inside me was gushing out in what seemed like an endless torrent. With each spasm of my cock, she moaned again, as if my climax was all she cared about. I don't know whether she came or not, but when I was finished, she let out a long sigh as if she had just been to heaven. As we untangled our legs and arms and got up from the floor, I got the distinct impression our date was over.

I left Amy's place and walked about three miles to get home. There were buses running, but I wanted to walk and think. This was definitely the most exciting thing that ever happened to me—a million times sexier than the quickie on the rooftop. For one thing, there had been no exchange of money. That meant the girl was doing it for pleasure, and her pleasure consisted of getting me inside her and getting me off. Also, knowing that I was going to see her at the academy the next day and every day for a while after that was a tremendous turn-on. From that point on, every time I saw her, I would remember that fantastic fuck on her living room floor.

I knew that she went out with lots of guys at the academy, so I figured I had got lucky and wasn't expecting a repeat. Then, a couple of days after our date, she surprised me at lunchtime by asking me to check something out with her. She led me into this concrete building that we used for fire-fighting drills. The inside was blackened and charred from all the practice fires that had burned there. There was no furniture, nothing but bare walls. But that didn't stop her.

The instant we got into the shelter of the building, she unzipped my fly and took out my cock. It was already half hard, but she stroked it for a couple of seconds to make it harder. Then, without a word, she undid her own pants and dropped them, lifting one foot out of them so that they remained bunched around her other ankle.

She was wearing filmy pink panties. I remember thinking about how strange they looked under the sexless academy uniform. Without further ado, she took hold of the crotch-band and pulled it to one side, exposing the dense bush of black hair that surrounded her pussy. I got a look at the shiny pink lips and the swollen button of her clit, but not for long.

"Hurry," she said, "before somebody finds us here." With that, she pulled my cock toward her and inserted me deep inside her. As I felt the flesh of her pussy closing around me, the climax started rising in my balls. It was so warm and wet inside her. I wanted to be sure she got something out of it, too, so I tried to hold it back as long as I could.

She must have sensed that, because she said, "No, don't fight it. Come as fast as you can. Come in me. Come in me. Come in me. Come in me." It was like a song that she kept chanting, until her words combined with the sensations I was feeling to drive me right over the top. I couldn't have held back any longer if I tried. Anyway, by then I had quit trying.

I felt myself emptying into her, filling her with gallons of my hot foam. Just as she had on the floor of her apartment, she moaned and sobbed with each spurt, as if she was experiencing my orgasm with me. That excited me almost as much as the fuck itself. I just kept on coming.

Finally, when I was spent, my cock started going limp and sort of popped out of her, followed by a stream of hot juice. She asked for my handkerchief, which she used to wipe herself with, and then handed it back to me, saying, "Here's a souvenir. I'll see you in class."

She was gone before I finished dressing. I couldn't help thinking that here was a woman I had fucked twice, and yet I had never seen or felt her titties. Somehow, that became a special turn-on. It made the experience feel just like that first time on the roof.

I went out with Amy a few more times after that. Our dates always ended with a fast, down-and-dirty fuck. At first, there was always some reason to hurry, some possibility of getting caught. Later, there was a couple of times when we were perfectly safe, and yet she still wanted it quick and without ceremony. Truth is, I never did get to see her tits. When our course at the academy ended, Amy and myself went our separate ways.

A few years later, after I had been working as a fireman for a while, I met Norma. We dated for quite some time before we started having sex. By then, she had managed to let me know that sex and romance were all tied together in her mind. She would no more think of having sex with someone she didn't love than she would fuck on a roof, standing up.

It wasn't until after she was sure that we were committed to each other that she let me touch her in a sexual way. For weeks, all I got to do was feel her breasts. We'd spend hours sitting on a sofa kissing and cuddling. My hands would roam over the front of her blouse and sometimes my fingers would sneak inside it. It seemed like ages before she let me remove her blouse and bra, and lots more time went by before I could get any further than that.

The first time we actually made love took about three hours from start to finish. After all that, it was very rewarding to hear her cries of ecstasy. A whole different experience than the quickies I had experienced before.

I took pride in bringing Norma to climax, knowing that her standards were high and figuring I must be a pretty powerful dude if I could satisfy her. That pride sustained me for the first three or four years of our marriage. But lately, there are times when I find myself dreading the whole sex ordeal.

Sometimes, I come home from work so tired and hungry that all I want is a fast fuck before dinner. Unfortunately, that's never the way it is with us. For Norma, sex always has to be a big production. It seems like I have to work so hard at turning her on that I don't get to enjoy it the way I'd like to.

Now, I'm not saying that I want it like that all the time. Just once in a while, it would be nice to get fast relief with my wife. To me, I guess that still seems like the most exciting kind of sex there is. I can't see that happening, though. At least not now. Sometimes I'm tempted to pick up a hooker or something, just to get a chance to indulge this secret desire of mine. I won't, of course. I'd never cheat on my wife.

I doubt if I'll ever tell her about my need. Even if I did, I doubt she'd go along with it. I'll just have to content myself with old memories and dreams about quickies. Maybe when your book is published, I can give it to her as a present. Maybe it'll help her get the idea.

Shameful Fantasy

$\mathscr{M}$ary, thirty-nine, is the owner of a small string of boutiques, having built her business from the bottom up by hard work and ingenuity. She is of medium height and thin, but with sensuous curves. Her dark brown hair is cut short, with streaks of gray that give her a quiet air of dignity. Her bright blue eyes flash as she talks of her humble beginnings.

My parents died when I was only seven years old. I was brought up by nuns in a convent. They were loving, but strict, and taught all of us girls a very rigid system of morality. I remember, even at that young age, that they told us that when we went to sleep, God wanted us to keep our hands on top of the blankets. I didn't understand then why God would care about where I kept my hands. I realize now it was to keep us from touching ourselves while we lay in our beds.

I don't ever remember their talking directly about sex. I do know I grew up believing that outside of marriage, it was a terrible thing. Even within marriage, it was questionable unless it was specifically aimed at reproduction. I kept to that belief until I was well into adulthood. To this day, I have never even masturbated.

Somewhere along the line, I realized that sex was a necessary part of life, whether a person is married or not. I guess I learned that from Claude. I met him in the business world, a good ten years ago. At first, our relationship was strictly business. After a year or two, we began to build up a different kind of friendship.

Claude is considerably older than I am. He has been married for a very long time. His wife has been disabled for years and spends most of her life in institutions. There are times when she doesn't even recognize him. Then there are times when she seems to live just for his visits. Claude is very loyal to her and would never think of leaving her or divorcing her. First of all, he's Catholic, like me. Second of all, he feels a strong sense of obligation to her.

One evening, we were talking about it over dinner. He confessed that the total lack of sex was driving him crazy. I was a little shocked to hear him speaking that way, but as I thought about it, I realized that the needs that were satisfied during the earlier part of his marriage did not go away just because his wife was ill. That got me thinking about my own life. Although I was in my twenties, I had never had sexual contact of any kind, not even with myself.

I don't exactly know how it happened, but little by little our relationship became more intimate. Soon I was telling him about my sexual ignorance and confessing my curiosity. Let's face it, at that point in my life, it was more than idle curiosity. I was a normal, healthy woman, with a normal, healthy woman's needs and desires. I had just been suppressing them.

One night, after dinner, I found myself in a hotel room with Claude and in his arms. We kissed long and passionately. Believe it or not, it was my very first kiss. A lot of firsts happened that night.

While we were kissing, his hands moved to my breasts and to my bottom, caressing me hungrily through my clothes. I realized that we were going to end up making love. I felt my face turning red at the thought of it. It went against everything I had been taught, but I wanted it to happen more than anything else in the world.

I've read that women seldom have orgasms during their first sexual experience. I guess mine was an exception.

Claude was slow and patient, leading me through all the steps to full and complete arousal. He seemed to place his own needs in the background and cater only to mine. He undressed me slowly and touched me everywhere. First he stroked me and then he kissed and nibbled at me. By the time he began removing his own clothes, I was feverish with desire.

Our bodies were nude and pressed tightly together when he entered me. I was expecting a searing pain, but felt only a mild discomfort as he worked himself in. Then my body went wild. I wrapped my arms and legs around him and gave myself to him completely. I think I screamed when the orgasm overtook me. It was my very first and totally indescribable.

My relationship with Claude changed after that. In addition to the deep mutual respect that we felt for each other, there was also passion. He was patient with me, a gentleman at all times. We began getting together two nights a week, always finishing the evening in bed. I knew I could count on lovemaking that would go on for hours at a time.

He satisfied all my yearnings. Well, almost all. There were times I wished he would just mount me and take me. Quickly and roughly. Use me like a toy and then put his pants back on. Then, maybe later, he could make patient love to me.

Although I had not quite gotten over the belief that sex outside of marriage would lead to damnation, I thought our affair was justified by the respect that we felt for each other. Allowing myself to be taken without emotion would have been different. That truly would have been sinful. Maybe that's why the idea appealed to me so.

I didn't feel I could tell Claude about it, for a few reasons. First, I appreciated the patience and consideration he showed me during our lovemaking. I couldn't have said anything that might make him think there was anything about it that disappointed me. Then, I don't think a woman ought to be sexually aggressive. Telling him what to do or how to make love would have crossed that line. It would have made me feel whorish. Finally, I knew that he, too, was a religious person. I was afraid that if he knew I even harbored such a desire, he would see me in a different light. He would think I was unworthy of him, unworthy of any love or respect at all.

So I buried my secret hunger. Which may account for how I got involved with Devon. I hate to admit this, but my attraction to him was purely physical at first. At some level of my consciousness, I think I saw him as the man who could fulfill my secret fantasy about being roughly and hurriedly taken.

I had won the door prize at a business dinner I attended. It turned out to be a short cruise on one of those gambling ships. I don't gamble—another lesson I learned early in life—but I was looking forward to a few days of sunshine and relaxation. Honestly, that's all I had in mind.

The second day aboard, I was stretched out on a deck chair, enjoying the gentle rocking of the ocean, when a burly, powerful-looking man dropped into the chaise next to mine. He began talking immediately, as if we already knew each other. "Well, you seem to know what a cruise is for," he began, in a very friendly voice.

My first instinct was to ignore him, but there was something about his obvious strength that appealed to me. He didn't look like the typical cruise ship passenger, so I wasn't surprised when he told me that he worked on the ship. When he said that, I pictured him hauling up an anchor or swabbing down a deck. It turned out he was a cook in the ship's galley. We talked for a while, until he announced that he had to go back to work. Almost shyly, he asked if he could see me later. Casually, I agreed to meet him at the same place about an hour after dinner.

For the rest of the afternoon, my mind reeled with sexual fantasies. The thought of making love to a sailor, even a ship's cook, had a strange kind of mystery for me. I imagined his body, covered with hair and tattoos from ports of call all over the world. His muscles would ripple as he would tear my clothes off and throw me down to the floor or onto a swinging hammock to plunge into me.

I pictured it over and over again, in many different ways, but always abrupt and swift. Each time my mind conjured up an image of such unceremonious sex, I would be overwhelmed by a sense of guilt accompanied by an unbelievable stimulation. I could feel my underwear getting tight and uncomfortable at the thought of being taken at the whim of this powerful denizen of the seas. I realized that only a loose woman would feel that way. That filled me with shame, but not enough to abolish my fantasies.

By the time dinner was over, I was primed and ready for a sexual adventure. I couldn't believe that, after speaking to this man for less than an hour, I was all set to have sex with him. But I was; there was no doubt about it.

When we met as planned, I couldn't even concentrate on our conversation. He was dressed in tight white pants and an even tighter T-shirt, with horizontal stripes that emphasized his strength. All I could think of was being swept up into his arms and carried off to be used as a sexual toy. I don't know how it happened, but we ended up rushing to my stateroom together.

I held my breath as we entered and the door closed behind us. I was certain that he would get rough now, that his brutal sexuality would get the best of him, that I would be victimized by his unbridled hunger for my body. I was fully prepared to surrender, to be taken without preamble, to be a pawn in his erotic game. That wasn't the way it happened.

Instead, he murmured, "Oh, how exciting it is to be alone with you," taking me gently into his arms. "I want to please you," he crooned. "I want to make you feel so good. From the very first sight that my eyes took hold of you, I felt a thunderbolt within me."

Nobody had ever talked to me that way before. Although Claude and I enjoyed a real friendship and mutual respect, there had never been talk of deep attraction or of thunderbolts. Claude was older and more reserved. Devon's eyes flashed in a way Claude's never could. I was flattered and, in a way, honored by his attention.

He started kissing me and I yielded completely to him. Gone for the moment was all thought of being taken roughly and hungrily, of being used and abused. Devon was a skillful lover, lifting me to heights of excitement that I had never experienced before. He did things to me with his lips and tongue that Claude had never done. Things that I never thought would ever happen to me.

He seduced my body for a long time, leading me slowly along the gently winding path of sexual arousal. When, at last, I reached the top of the mountain, my release seemed the most comfortable and natural thing in the world. I just let it go, feeling the waves of orgasmic satisfaction washing over me until I was completely relaxed and fulfilled. Only then did Devon allow himself to climax, moaning hoarsely as the paroxysms of pleasure heaved through him and into me.

Afterwards, we lay together in each other's arms, absorbing the warmth and softness of our experience. It was the first time in my life I had felt what it was like to be loved. Early in the morning, Devon slipped out of my room, returning a few minutes later with a tray from the galley, covered with delicacies and treats that the rest of the passengers rarely got to see.

He left me to breakfast alone because he had to go to work, but we got together later that afternoon and again that evening. Both times, we made fantastic love, each session more beautiful and satisfying than the last. When the cruise ended, he took my phone number and promised to call me.

I've been seeing Devon regularly since then, every two or three weeks, whenever his cruise ship is in port. It's hard to believe that a girl with my background has two lovers, but I do. So far, there haven't been any conflicts. My nights with Claude never seem to coincide with the times when Devon's in town. There are times I feel guilty about it. Yet I like them both so much, in two different ways, that I could never think of giving either of them up.

I really wish one of them, either of them, would stop being so considerate and patient, even if only for one night. I still have fantasies about being thrown down and taken roughly. It doesn't look like those fantasies will ever come true. Maybe it's the guilt that makes me feel that way.

Maybe, deep down, I feel that a woman who behaves as I do ought to be mistreated by men, ought to be used for their pleasure without any regard for her own. I don't know what the reason is. I just know I'd like to experience it. I've never told this to anybody before. I know I'll never tell Claude or Devon. But it sure felt good to tell you.

TWO

The Sex Business

$\mathcal{A}$n old song says, "I work eight hours. I sleep eight hours. That leaves eight hours for fun." Nowadays, the arithmetic does not always work out so happily. In order to work eight hours, most of us spend one to three hours commuting. Some even have second jobs. When we get home, we have kids to feed and other household responsibilities. Few people sleep a full eight hours every night. Most have very little time for fun.

Since such a large fraction of life is work-related, it is not surprising to hear of people for whom sexuality and business are closely linked. Some dream of actually being in the sex business. Others imagine ways of bringing sex into what ever business they happen to be in. This chapter gives three examples.

Roberta, a massage therapist, fantasizes about sex while practicing her profession. Eugene, a real estate broker, reminisces about the career as a porno star at which he almost, but never really, had a chance. Tonya wishes she were a call girl, using her imagination to escape from an existence that she finds miserable and oppressive. For each of them, the fantasy is as far away from the reality of life as it could possibly be. Is it any wonder that their desires remain unspoken?

Massage

*A*t forty-eight, Roberta is tall and stocky, with broad, muscular shoulders and powerful arms. Her eyes, like her hair, are steely gray. Her bosom is large, her body narrowing only slightly at her thick waist, flaring out again to wide hips. Heavy but well-proportioned thigh muscles ripple under the white uniform skirt that she wears. Roberta's hands and fingers are almost masculine in their obvious strength. She is a massage therapist.

You'd better disguise my identity real good. I have a great job and I wouldn't want to lose it. I'm a staff body-worker at one of the best health clubs in the city. We have a contract with a professional basketball team that really keeps me busy. Not only do I get paid for each massage I give, but I get tips besides, and sometimes that's even more than the salary. At Christmas, the gifts from satisfied clients really mount up.

I don't really know why I'm telling you this, except that it's on my mind so much. I've never been able to tell anybody else. For one thing, it's supposed to be highly unprofessional to have thoughts like these. If my husband, Dale, knew about it, I think he'd be so shocked that he'd make me quit my job.

I've received years of training and I've had more years of experience. I have a tremendous respect for the human body—temple of the soul, and all that. But I must admit that sometimes when I get a guy laid out on a table and begin working on him, I get fascinated by the sight of his dick.

Most of the men I work on are big and tall. Somehow their sex organs always seem to be in proportion to the rest of their body. There's one in particular who's almost seven feet tall and has a dick that stretches practically to his knee. I try hard not to notice it, but that's almost impossible.

When I received my training, I was taught that the client should always be partially covered with a sheet. Some teachers said he should be completely covered, except for whatever part we happened to be working on. Others said only the genitals had to be kept covered, since we would never be touching him there. Over the years, I've found that I can give a better massage if I dispense with the sheet all together.

For one thing, that eliminates the need to keep fooling around with it, draping and redraping the client as I move around his body. For another, there are times when I do come awfully close to the genitals, especially when working on an athlete. They tend to get painful knots high up on the thigh, sometimes in that crease where the thigh meets the torso. If I had to worry about a sheet all the time, the massage would take twice as long, and the flow would be constantly interrupted. I know I'm not gorgeous. Maybe it's my looks that keep the men from feeling embarrassed about being totally naked in front of me. Ah, it would be different if they knew what I was thinking.

I only actually behaved unprofessionally one time, and that was back in massage school. Our instructor had divided us into teams. We were supposed to practice on each other. My partner—let's just call him John—was a hulk of a man, but I remember thinking maybe he was gay. Anyway, he was lying on a table and I was working on him, when I decided to find out.

Teasingly, almost accidentally, I let the tips of my fingers stroke through his pubic hair and brush against the little spot where his scrotum met his penis. I saw an instant response. Just a kind of shudder that seemed to go through his genitals. When I touched him there again, his dick stood up straight and hard. Without even thinking about it, I wrapped my hand around it and began stroking up and down.

His breathing became heavy and labored, his eyes shut tight, and his muscles all went rigid. Then, with a gasp, his dick began to swell and his belly began to ripple, as the first spurt of his orgasm came shooting out. It all happened so fast that I didn't even appreciate what I had done until it was over. Then I found my hands, his belly, and the table covered with the sticky substance. Using a hot towel, I quickly cleaned up. I found it awfully hard to look him in the eye.

We never spoke about it after that. Coincidentally, our instructor rearranged the teams the following day, and I was paired with another woman. I always wondered if John had anything to do with it.

For years, I managed to put that incident out of my mind, writing it off to immaturity and a beginner's mistake. But lately, I find the memory creeping back into my consciousness whenever I get one of those basketball players on my table. You can't imagine how magnificent these men look and what an effect they have on me.

I think of how it would be to touch their dicks to make them stand up straight and tall like John's did that afternoon at the school. My head is filled with thoughts of all the erotic things I could do if I weren't so inhibited. I'd like to run the tips of my fingers up and down the length of some of those statuesque penises, feeling the swelling muscles under the surface, sensing the coursing blood through the engorged vessels, twirling my hands over the velvety purple tips.

Many of my clients are black men, and their dicks sometimes look like polished ebony. I even imagine bending over and stroking them with my lips and tongue. I would take as much of the stiff dick into my mouth as I possibly could, massaging it with the insides of my cheeks. Then, when it was wet with a mixture of my saliva and the gooey substance that oozed from it, I would take it in my hand again and stroke it softly but firmly, caressing it in a way that no vagina possibly could.

I would stretch out the process so that it would take a long time for him to reach an orgasm. Then, just as I sensed he was about to begin, I'd slow down and squeeze his shaft to stop it from happening. When his dick was half soft, I'd begin the whole routine again. Maybe I'd keep stroking him until his juices flew through the air and splashed on his belly. Or maybe I'd take him back in my mouth and suck on him until I felt him emptying himself down my throat. Then when it was over, I'd rub him softly all over with a warm towel, and calm him back to reality.

Can you realize how it is for me to have my hands on a naked athlete with a near-perfect body and all the time to be thinking about rubbing his dick? Sometimes, it gets me so stimulated that I feel myself becoming wet between the legs. Once in a while, I have to go into the ladies' room to relieve myself with my fingers.

Sometimes I give Dale a personal massage at home. I have a portable table, which I set up in our bedroom. Little does he realize that the best massages he ever gets are after I've had one of my fantasy experiences with one of my athletes. Usually, my touch becomes so sensual that Dale gets an erection almost immediately and retains it throughout the entire massage.

I'd love to grab it and stroke it and suck on it the way I've imagined doing with the basketball players. I don't, though, because I don't want him to associate sex with my work. I guess I'm afraid that if I start massaging his sex organs, he'll think I'm doing the same to my clients, or at least he'll suspect that I'm thinking about it. So I guess this will have to remain a secret desire of mine. Nothing but a fantasy.

Porno Star

At forty-four, Eugene has gray hair gray, almost white. Contrasted with his dazzling green eyes, it tends to give him a handsome, distinguished look. He is six feet three inches tall, with a lean and muscular body that shows traces of the wonderful physique he must have had when he was a youth. He speaks with a friendly manner that helps to account for his success as a real estate broker.

I spend a lot of time sitting on my butt these days, but when I was a younger man, I was a real Hercules. I worked out with weights three or four times a week and concentrated on sculpting my body to the perfection of a Greek god. Nowadays, they do it with steroids. I did it with sweat and good hard work. For relaxation, I played basketball, handball, and all the other vigorous sports. You might say I was into the body culture.

That's probably what led to my relationship with Jill. I was working in the warehouse of a supermarket chain. I guess I was eighteen or nineteen. Jill was my supervisor, even though she was only a couple of years older than me.

I was eating lunch all by myself in the employee lounge when Jill walked in. She looked quickly around and said, "I'm glad I found you here alone." I was expecting to get bawled out for something I had done or not done on the job. After all, she was my boss. Until that day she had never spoken to me about anything at all but work. She surprised me, though.

"I've got a proposition for you," she said. "It could change your whole life."

Let me stop for a minute and tell you about this gal. She was too damn good-looking to be working in a supermarket warehouse. She was tall and shapely, with big tits and a firm round ass that could stop your heart from beating. She had jet-black hair that hung almost to her waist when it wasn't tucked under a hard hat. Her eyes were so brown they were almost black.

The guys all talked about her when she wasn't around. Every one of them would have given whatever it took to get into her bed. There was something so regal and aloof about her that she seemed totally unapproachable.

Naturally, I was all ears when she said the word "proposition." Not even my wildest fantasies would have prepared me for what came next. "I've had an offer to audition for a movie," she said.

"Congratulations," I answered, a little puzzled about why she was telling this to me. "I always thought you were star material. I hope you make it. Send me a postcard from Hollywood."

"Well," she began, with a shyness that seemed out of character. "It isn't exactly a Hollywood movie."

It was obvious that I was expected to ask, so I did. "What kind of movie is it?"

She looked around the room again, as if to make sure that no one had come in without being heard. "It's a porno flick," she said in a husky voice that was just above a whisper. I didn't know what to say to that, so I said nothing. She continued, "They asked me to bring a male partner, and I thought of you immediately. With your build and your good looks, you'd be a natural."

I was so bewildered that I was speechless. She looked at me, waiting for my response. I just didn't know how to answer. "Well," she prodded. "Are you interested?"

I would have gone along with the scheme just for the

chance of getting next to Jill. On top of that, the idea of being in porno movies was my favorite fantasy. Shit, let's face it, at that age, it's every young man's fantasy. And who could have asked for a better partner.

"Yeah, I'm interested," I said enthusiastically. "This is kind of sudden and a little hard to digest. Let me understand something. What is it exactly that I . . . er, you and I . . . er, we . . . will be expected to do?"

"Just what you think," she said. "If you're willing, I'll call them back and make an appointment for the audition. Then we go to their studio, I guess, and we perform."

"Aah, that's the part I'm wondering about," I asked uncomfortably. "What do you mean by 'perform'?"

"We have sex, I guess," she answered. She seemed as uncertain as I. "We do whatever they tell us to do. You can be sure that sex is going to be part of it. Is that okay with you?"

It sure was. I could feel myself blushing. I knew nothing about Jill's personal life, but I certainly never thought she would be this casual about sex. In an attempt to cover up, I asked, "Do we have to learn any lines or anything?"

"I don't think so," she said. "I'm sure they'll give me the details when I call."

"And we get paid for this?" I asked, unable to hide my amazement.

"Well, not for the audition," she explained. "If they use us in a movie, they'll be paying us plenty. You know how it is in movies. If you're popular with the public, they use you again and again and again."

I wasn't just going to be in a porno movie. I was going to be a porno star. My god, who could have asked for more? "When can you call them?" I inquired anxiously.

She said she'd call right then, from her office, and get back to me in the lounge. I said I'd wait, trying to sound nonchalant. Shit, it would have taken a team of twenty mules to drag me out of there.

She was back a few minutes later. "It's all set," she said.

"We're meeting them Friday night at eight. I'll arrange the schedule so we can leave here at seven-thirty. We'll go together."

Friday was two whole days away. I didn't know how I would survive until then. My mind was spinning with pornographic images. While waiting for the big day to come, I thought about Jill all the time. Whenever I saw her on the floor of the warehouse, I realized that I was soon going to be naked with her and having sex with her. I might be eating her. She might be eating me. Surely we'd be fucking. I just couldn't believe it.

Even more exciting than that was the thought of getting into porno movies. That meant unlimited sex partners. Best of all, I wouldn't have to lift a finger to get them. The movie producers would be matching me up with some of the most beautiful women in the world, two and three at a time, just so we could fuck in front of the camera. The sex would be boundless.

Knowing that there would be a camera did give me some tense moments. Once I was on film, it would be permanent. I sure wouldn't have wanted anyone I knew to see and recognize me in one of those movies. But I didn't really know anyone who went to the sleazy porno theaters that existed at the time.

I don't think VCRs had been invented yet. At any rate, nobody had one. I never imagined there would soon be one in every American household, or that sex movies would be available on the shelves of video stores for a couple of bucks a night. Besides, a young man's hormones are stronger than his reason. The prospect of all that free-flowing sex overpowered any sense of caution I might have had.

By the time Friday came around, my powerful young body was like a tower of Jell-O. I was trembling and shaking all over. When I saw Jill in the warehouse, we both tried to act natural so that the other workers wouldn't suspect anything. I could see she was every bit as nervous as I was.

At seven-thirty we left the warehouse separately to meet

in the parking lot. I didn't have a car at the time, so we got into Jill's station wagon. We hardly spoke as she drove through the city streets. Finally, I asked, "Where is the studio?"

"We're not going to their studio," she answered. "This is only an audition. They said that the studio setting might make us too nervous to perform. So they suggested a hotel. We're meeting them at the Rockford, uptown." I had never been there, but I recognized the name. It was one of the fanciest hotels around.

When we got there, we stopped at the desk and asked for Mr. Moore's room, as Jill had been instructed to do. The desk clerk phoned and, after getting permission, gave us the room number and told us to go on up. In the elevator, we were both too nervous to speak.

The room turned out to be a luxurious suite. We were greeted at the door by an attractive woman somewhere in her late forties. She was dressed very expensively, and her hair was elegantly coifed. "I'm Mrs. Moore," she said. "This is my husband, Mr. Moore." A man in a finely tailored suit stepped forward and shook Jill's hand and mine, making a little bow as he did. "It's our film you'll be auditioning for," he explained.

We tried to relax on couches in the sitting room. They offered us wine, which we readily accepted. By the third glass, I was feeling a little less tense. I could sense that Jill was calmer, too.

After some small talk, Mrs. Moore said, "Well, let's get started. We aren't going to give you a script to work from or tell you what we want you to do. We're most interested in how natural you are having sex. So we'll just ask you to undress each other and proceed as if we weren't here. Shall we go into the bedroom?"

Silently, Jill and I followed the couple into another room. In it was a king-sized bed with the covers removed., Beside the bed were a pair of easy chairs. The Moores sat in them, and Mrs. said, "All right, now. Go ahead."

I started to undress Jill very slowly, admiring the way she looked at each stage of the process. When she was down to bra and panties, I began kissing all the skin that was exposed, from her thighs and belly to the roundness of her breasts where they swelled out from the top of her bra. I started to unhook it, but she stopped me and began undressing me. When she had me down to my shorts, she kissed me all over, the way I had been kissing her.

The nervousness passed at once. We became two young people driven by lust. I removed her underwear and she removed mine. I played with her breasts, cupping them and stroking the erectness of her brown nipples. She took my stiff cock in her hand and rubbed it gently, making it quiver with excitement.

I lay her down on the bed and began licking her body everywhere, working my way toward her groin. When I arrived, I began tonguing her vagina, rolling her swollen clit around in my mouth, and nibbling on the tender, sweet-tasting flesh of her insides. I could taste the fluids of her excitement flowing under my plunging tongue.

After a while, we switched roles and she went down on me, taking my cock into her mouth and swabbing it lightly with strokes of her tongue as her head bobbed up and down. Her hands cupped my scrotum, rolling my balls around as she ate me. It took all my strength to keep from coming in her mouth, but I knew that my career in porno films depended on this performance. That helped me hold back.

We climbed on top of each other and sixty-nined. I tasted her sex at the same time that she tasted mine. I could feel her throat opening to accept the head of my cock. It was the best oral sex I had ever experienced, either as giver or receiver. Soon, we both forgot that anyone but us was in the room.

I could hear the sounds Jill was making as she devoured my cock. They were mingled with moans that my ministrations were bringing from her throat. I knew I was pleasing her. That turned me on even more.

Letting my cock slip from her mouth, Jill murmured, "Oh, Eugene, I want to fuck you." She rolled over and climbed on top of me, mounting me and reaching down with her hand to insert my bucking hard-on into her warm and well-lubricated channel. When it was inside, I lifted my hips and drove myself up as deep as I could.

She rode me while I held her voluminous breasts with both my hands. I rolled her nipples in my fingers and stroked her massive, magnificent curves. I could see an expression of rapture on her face. Her eyes were closed tightly. Her mouth was slightly open, as if it was a struggle for her to get enough air.

We kept it up for a long time, rolling over so that I was on top of her, and then rolling back so that she was on top of me again. When she was on the bottom, she lifted her legs high into the air, pointing her toes at the ceiling, before clenching her thighs around my waist. When she was on top, she rolled her ass down hard against me, forcing me all the way inside her.

At last, writhing under me, she gasped and whispered, "I can't hold back any longer. I'm going to come." I had been fighting it for so long that all it took were her words to rob me of all strength.

As the first wave of climax rolled over her, I began to explode. Quickly, I pulled my squirting penis from inside her. With one hand, I rubbed her clitoris. With the other, I stroked my cock, aiming it at her heaving breasts, as the men did in every porno movie I had ever seen. She seemed to like it, because each time a spurt hit her, she moaned a little louder. When our orgasms were completed, I fell forward on top of her and kissed her on the lips.

After a few minutes, Mr. and Mrs. Moore got out of their chairs and stood by the side of the bed. "Very nice," she said. "That will be all for now. We'll go into the other room to give you a chance to get dressed."

When we went into the living room, they handed us our coats and she said, "We'll be in touch." I had the feeling they were hustling us out of the suite. I thought maybe we had excited them to the point where they wanted to be alone for a little action of their own. Or that maybe they were expecting another couple for an another audition.

In the car, Jill and I chattered incessantly about how our screentest went. She kept saying, "I'm sure they were impressed. I know I was. You're a wonderful lover. We're going to be in the movies. We're going to make a lot of money starring in porno films."

A few weeks went by, but we received no word from the Moores. Finally, I asked Jill to call them. She said she was too nervous and gave me their card. So I called them.

Mrs. Moore gave me some bullshit in the language of the day. If it had been now, she would have been saying something like, "We have decided to abandon the project." The bottom line was, no film career. Later, I realized that there never was a porno movie in the making. It was just a scam they used to watch a good-looking young couple having sex. I was disappointed.

Some good came out of it, though. Jill and I had a torrid affair that lasted until she met her present husband and got engaged to marry him. In that time, we became good friends. Even today, she's still one of my very best friends. She and her husband get together with me and my wife every couple of weeks, and sometimes more often than that.

Of course, if my wife knew what Jill and I experienced that Friday night in a bedroom at the Rockford Hotel, she'd probably never want to see her again. That would end our friendship. I sure wouldn't want to risk that happening. Which is one reason why my abortive career in the porno industry is something I'll never be able to tell my wife about.

Rim Artist

onya is twenty-two years old. Her fingers and teeth are already yellow with nicotine stains. There appears to be a trace of a homemade tattoo on the back of her left hand, which she has a tendency to hide as she speaks. She is very thin, with stringy blond hair and pale, almost sickly, white skin. Her shoulders and hips are narrow, her breasts boyishly small. She cups the tiny cones in her hands for a moment through her stained shirt as she starts speaking.

I may not look like much, now, but I'll bet I'd clean up real good. I was pretty as a kid. All the guys wanted me. Most of them had me. Until Henri came along and ruined my life.

Henri's my husband, and he don't know a fucking thing about me. If it wasn't for him, I might of been able to make something out of myself. I'm only with him because of my daughter, Connie. I don't intend to be with him too much longer. I've just got to find a way out of here. I'd make one hell of a call girl. But it takes money to get started in something like that.

I always liked sex, ever since I was a little girl. I played sex games with all my friends until I started developing. Then I was ready for the real thing. By the time I was thirteen I was already fucking and sucking. Sometimes with guys my own age; sometimes with older guys—sixteen, seventeen, like that.

I must of been real good at it, because word got around

the neighborhood. There was always somebody calling me up and wanting to fuck me. It made me feel important.

I loved the way I could make a guy whimper like a baby just by stroking his cock or letting him touch my pussy. I'll never forget, I brought tears to one guy's eyes by licking his asshole. A rimjob he'll remember for the rest of his life.

When I met Henri, I was seventeen. He was one of the guys I'd seen around the neighborhood. He belonged to a little gang and walked tough all the time. One day, he saw me sitting on the stoop in front of the building I lived in and came up to me. "Hey, girl," he said. "Wanna go for a ride on my motorcycle."

"Sure," I said, always up for a new adventure. Not many of the kids in my neighborhood had wheels of their own, so the thought of being seen on the back of his bike was pretty hot. A couple minutes later we was tearing up and down the streets, turning heads and feeling the wind in our faces. A few minutes after that, we pulled up in front of an old abandoned building about eight blocks away from where I lived.

Henri got off the bike and wheeled it with him as he led me into the building. "Ain't gonna leave it out here," he said. "Sure as shit, somebody would steal it."

I followed him into the building's dark basement, half wondering what was coming next, and half already knowing. When we got down there, he leaned the motorcycle against a wall and grabbed me into his arms. He started kissing me. I kissed back, sticking my tongue deep into his throat. Pretty soon, he had me naked and was fucking me right there on the floor. No fooling around for Henri. He just got right down to business.

All of the other guys I fucked had enough sense to use condoms. But Henri was too macho for that. I tried to say something about it, but he pressed his lips tight against mine to shut me up. Then he said, "Don't worry; I'll pull out."

That first fuck was over in a few seconds. He pulled out like he said he would, and I felt his cum going all over my legs. Then we got dressed and went for another ride on his bike. Later that afternoon, a couple of my girlfriends told me they were pretty impressed to see me with him. That was all I had to hear.

I kept seeing Henri after that, more for the prestige than anything else. It sure wasn't for the sex. I mean, his idea of fucking was stick it in, pull it out, shoot all over me, and put his clothes back on. Far as he was concerned, I had no needs of my own. Or if I did, they didn't matter worth a shit.

I was still fucking some other guys, and Henri knew it. He didn't seem to care as long as he got his. But then the shit hit the fan. I missed a period. And then another one. When I started feeling sick in the mornings, I knew I had to be pregnant. I knew it was Henri's, 'cause he was the only one who did it without a condom.

After a while, I told him, figuring maybe he could come up with some money for an abortion. He shocked me by saying, "Fuck. Now we gotta get married." I didn't want to marry him or anybody else at that point. I was barely eighteen. But he absolutely would not hear of an abortion. It was his kid, he said, and he was going to do the right thing.

Next thing I knew, we were talking to the priest. He also thought we should get married immediately, before my belly started to swell. So we did. One morning, me and Henri met at the church and said the words. My mother was there, but my father couldn't make it. Nobody from Henri's side was there.

After the ceremony, we went to Henri's apartment. It was empty. He told me that his father was long gone and his mother was in jail on a drug thing, so we'd have the place to ourselves for a few months. Well, it's been a few years and we still have it to ourselves. Only now we got Connie with us.

I'm crazy about Connie. Henri is too. It's the only thing decent about him. He went and got a job as a motorcycle mechanic and works hard to pay the rent and put food on the table. But he still don't give a shit about me.

When he comes home from work at night, he's tired and

he just flops down in front of the TV with Connie on his lap. He waits for me to serve him dinner, plays with her a little, then goes back to the TV and usually falls asleep in his chair. I haven't had a good fuck since I found out I was pregnant. Henri and I hardly ever do it at all. When we do, it's the same old stuff—stick it in, pull it out, come all over me, roll over, and go to sleep.

It's just as well. I find him disgusting. The creases in his fingers are always filled with black motorcycle grease. His hands are rough and dirty. His touch positively turns me off. Sometimes, I dream about the guys I used to fuck in the old neighborhood. None of them were a great lover, but at least they thought about someone besides themself.

If I could break away from this, though, I know exactly what I would do. I'd set myself up in a fancy apartment somewhere, maybe on the East Side. I'd furnish it in red velvet and other stuff that says sex, sex, sex. Maybe get some sexy pictures to hang on the walls. I'd fix myself up. Get my hair done. My nails. Get some of that underwear that would make my titties look bigger.

Then I'd start entertaining businessmen. I haven't forgotten how to give a good fuck, even if I've only been doing it in my head. In fact, I've remembered and imagined so many incidents, that I'm sure I'd be better than I ever was. I think a call girl ought to specialize in something. I'd specialize in rimjobs, you know, licking a guy's asshole.

Not many girls are even willing to do rimjobs. Those that do don't do them as good as me. I could really get into it. That would be my specialty. I'd be known far and wide as a rim artist.

Word would get around, and I'd be in a lot of demand. One night, a guy would call and say he came all the way from the West Coast to do it with me. I'd make an appointment for him to come up to my place. I'd meet him at the door in a sexy see-through negligee. I'd see him staring at my nipples and my pussy hair and I'd see his cock getting hard inside his pants.

His night would just be beginning. I'd be ready to give him the time of his life. He'd ask me to take off the negligee so he could see me totally naked. I'd do it and then turn slowly in place for him, so he could look at every part of me. I'd love the way it feels to have his eyes on my ass. Maybe I'd even bend over and hold my cheeks apart, so he could get a real good look at my asshole. That really turns some guys on.

Then I'd start undressing him. Real slow. First his jacket and tie. Then his shirt. Finally, I'd start working on his pants. He wouldn't be able to resist touching my titties and my pussy while I was doing this, but that would be all right with me. When I had his pants off, I'd see his cock sticking up hard through the fly of his shorts. As a sort of surprise, I'd bend over and start sucking on it. I'd love the sounds he'd make. Then I'd whip the shorts off him completely and have him as naked as I was.

I think it's important for a woman in the sex business to be in complete control. I would do everything to him that he'd want and expect, without him ever having to ask for it. The biggest, hottest part would be the rimjob. First I'd lay him on his back and kiss his whole body from head to feet. I'd trail my tongue over his nipples and spend a lot of time licking the wrinkled sack of his balls.

His cock would be jumping and twitching, like it was begging for a little suck, and I'd give it to him. I'd take that swollen rod all the way down my throat, massaging it by making swallowing motions. Then I'd keep on licking his thighs and legs until his whole body was shiny wet.

I'd turn him over then, and he'd know what was coming. I'd start nibbling the cheeks of his ass, using my fingers to spread them a little bit at a time. My tongue would slip between the cheeks and lap at the tight little bud of his asshole. All the while, I'd be listening to the sounds he'd be making. Moans. And groans. And heavy breathing.

Now my tongue would be making little circles around his asshole, each one bringing the tip closer and closer to the center. I can hear him sobbing like a baby. Then I slip my tongue inside the little hole, forcing the walls apart to make room for the plunge. Oh, he's practically crying now, digging the incredible sensation of having my tongue up his ass.

He starts humping up and down on the mattress, rubbing his cock against it as I buttfuck him with my tongue. I reach under him and cup his balls for a second before grabbing his cock. Now I'm jerking him off at the same time I'm reaming his asshole with my tongue. No man can stand much of that. I can feel his cock getting fatter and thicker as it fills with cum.

I might keep reaming him out while his cock spits onto the sheet. Or I might turn him over real quick and take his cock in my mouth while I shove a finger deep into his ass. If I really like the guy, I might straddle him and slip his cock into my pussy just in time for him to fill me with his cum. All the while, I'd be looking at the expression on his face and watching the distortions he'd be making as he'd be getting his rocks off.

When we were done, he'd be so satisfied that he'd give me twice as much as I usually charge. A couple of hundred bucks, for just having a good time in bed. Ah, that would be the life.

I'm telling you, I'd do it right now if I could just get out of here. First I'd have to get rid of Henri. Then I'd have to get some money. 'Cause apartments like that aren't cheap, and neither are the clothes. I've been having these dreams more and more often. I just know I'm getting closer to actually doing it. One day, real soon, I will. Then life will be something worth living.

THREE
Spice of Life

Society expects us to be monogamous—to go through life with only one sex partner. In this respect, homo sapiens come close to being unique. Very few life forms on this earth make any attempt at monogamy. In some other societies, and in some other times, no such expectation existed, even for humans. According to the Old Testament, for example, King Solomon had seven hundred wives and three hundred concubines.

We do not know whether monogamy is a natural state, or whether we have imposed it on ourselves for socio-religious reasons. We do know, however, that many people find it unsatisfying. Some resort to infidelity to satisfy their need for sexual variety. By entering into a series of marriages that all end in divorce, others engage in what some sociologists call serial polygamy.

We have interviewed many people who use fantasy to fulfill their longing for additional sex partners. This chapter presents two of their stories. Like Harry, some remember partners with whom they actually had sex at some time in the past. Others, like Lacey, imagine sex with someone with whom no actual contact ever occurred. Most of the time, they superimpose these imaginary or remembered encounters on sex with their spouses, keeping unspoken any desire they might have for real variety.

Neighbor

*L*acey, twenty-nine, has long, curly black hair and green eyes so bright that they seem to shine with their own inner light. She is about five feet eight inches tall, with the figure of a high-fashion model. In fact, she says she did some runway work when she was in her late teens. Her teeth are perfectly straight and white, a monument to cosmetic dentistry. Her smile is natural, though, and immediately gives a person the feeling that Lacey is comfortable with who she is. She carries a business card that lists her as a personal shopper, but she really doesn't need to work and spends most of her time lounging around her suburban southern California home.

Life is good here. My husband, Monte, has a very successful medical practice and I've gotten over the feeling that I had to make some kind of useful contribution to society. I like my leisure. Monte's income gives me the opportunity for plenty of it. Our daughter is only two, and I absolutely adore her, but our au pair takes care of her most of the time. So I am free to lie beside the pool, soaking up the sun and stealing glimpses of my neighbor, Rod.

Rod is a building contractor. In fact, he built our house. But that was before we owned it. He's done many of the custom homes in the area and has a reputation as a top-notch builder. Not that he does any of the building himself.

He's got lots of men working for him that do all the real

work. Rod leaves his house at about six-thirty every morning and spends a few hours visiting his many job sites and making sure his employees have their orders for the day. Then, about three-thirty he makes the rounds again to see how they've been progressing. In between, he just hangs around the house. Like I do.

His wife has some kind of a selling job and is away all day, but Rod doesn't seem to mind. He spends hours lying by his pool or swimming from one end to the other with long powerful strokes that make the sculptured muscles in his shoulders bulge. In looks, he's just the opposite of my husband.

Monte is the bookish type, kind of thin and pale, with eyes lost behind a pair of thick glasses in heavy black frames. His shoulders are narrow and his arms are on the skinny side. I don't mean to be putting him down. I love him. He's a good person and very considerate. We have a pretty good sex life, too.

But I'll never forget the first time I saw Rod. He's so handsome, I thought he might be a movie star. When a woman pictures having sex with the ideal partner, he's just the kind of guy she'd imagine. Tall. Dark wavy hair. Blue eyes that hypnotize you with one quick glance. And a flirty personality that seems to lure a woman into his inner world. He's eight or ten years older than me, about thirty-seven I'd guess.

Still, even though I admired his good looks, I don't think I ever thought about him in a sexual way until one afternoon when I was lying out by the pool. He came into his yard and stopped by the fence to call a greeting to me, as he frequently did. I sat up and smiled at him. I remember very clearly, I was wearing a tiny yellow bikini that covered nothing more than it was required to. He stood for a moment, his eyes roving freely over my body. His lips turned up in a contagious grin.

I didn't feel offended by the frankness of his gaze. In fact, I felt my body warming, as if I were being touched rather than just looked at. I was embarrassingly aware of my nipples beginning to harden inside the top of my suit, because I knew that their outline would be visible to him. When he saw them, he smiled even more broadly.

"Nice . . . er, bathing suit," he said, emphasizing the hesitation in a way that made it very intimate. I felt my face reddening. Funny, I thought I had outgrown blushing by the time I was seventeen, but there was something about him that made me feel girlish. I looked down to avoid his eyes and found myself looking at my own breasts, which made me even more flustered.

He laughed and said, "Well, see you later," plunging into the deep end of his pool, almost without a splash. As he swam underwater from one end to the other, I watched openly, admiring the way his muscular body moved. What a hunk. When he came up for air, he didn't even look in my direction. I was just too embarrassed by my own feelings to stay out there any longer. I went into the house and up to my bedroom.

That doesn't mean I stopped looking at him, though. In fact, I have a great view of his yard from my bedroom window. Maybe that's the real reason I went up there. As soon as I got into the room, I went to the window to watch him, knowing he wouldn't see me lurking there behind the curtains.

He was swimming rhythmically now, doing laps to keep his great body in great shape. I felt myself tingling all over, especially down there where my bikini bottom was clinging to my moistened crotch. I hadn't been in the water at all, but I was quite wet. I just stood there watching him.

I remember hoping deep inside that maybe, now that I was no longer in the yard, he would think he was alone and would take off his suit to swim nude. I had done it a couple of times, although only on dark nights. The idea apparently didn't even occur to him, so I had to content myself with imagining what he would look like in the nude.

The front of his tight swim suit appeared to be stuffed with some huge equipment. I think I was picturing an elephant's scrotum and a penis the size of a baseball bat. I imagined what it would look like if he slipped out of the suit and that huge organ sprang to erection before my eyes. The thought of it was making me wiggle a little, involuntarily, and the bottom of my bikini was starting to feel uncomfortable. Without taking my eyes off the sight of Rod swimming in his pool, I reached down and slipped my hand inside to feel the heat building in my vagina.

I was so wet that my fingers slid instantly between the lips and into the warm interior. Just like a teenager, I masturbated while watching my secret heartthrob without his knowledge. It only took a few moments for me to reach a climax. As I remember, it was a pretty good one. When it was finished, I felt a little foolish. I hadn't masturbated since I'd been married. I continued watching Rod for a while and then forced myself to turn away from the window and get dressed.

A few hours later, when Monte got home, I greeted him with a passionate embrace and whispered some sex talk in his ear. He usually has a drink as soon as he gets in, but this night I led him by the hand to the bedroom and undressed him while murmuring words of excitement. Within moments, we were both naked, rolling around on the bed. Monte always gives me good and thorough oral sex before penetrating me. That night, as usual, I lay back to enjoy it. As his lips and tongue moved over my heated membranes, all I could think of was Rod. Against my will, I imagined it was he doing all these things to me. I couldn't get his face and body out of my mind.

I was soon panting and moaning with excitement, letting Monte know that it was time to enter me. I closed my eyes tightly as he positioned himself between my thighs and began feeling for my opening with the tip of his penis. It was Rod's penis I was feeling and picturing, slowly spreading my vaginal lips to find its way into my sex.

By the time Monte got it in, I was so worked up that I wrapped my arms and legs around him and pulled him tight against me. I felt my fingernails ripping into the skin of his back, covering him with blood. My thighs crushed his waist as I raised my loins up against his penetrating thrusts. I was like a wild woman, fornicating for all I was worth.

I bit his lip with erotic abandon, tasting the salty flow of fresh blood. I screamed. I sobbed. I was totally out of control. By this time, so was Monte. His excitement was so elevated by my response that I could feel him throbbing and pulsating inside me. His breath was coming in hoarse gasps. All at once, a mutual orgasm was upon us. We climbed together to the pinnacle of erotic fulfillment and then coasted down the slope to contented calmness.

After we caught our breath, Monte said, "Wow, I've never, ever, seen you so hot. What aphrodisiac did you discover?" His words filled me with a sense of guilt. I'd been caught. He must have known what I'd been thinking. But then he said, "Whatever it is you've been smoking, please keep it up. I loved it."

For some time after that, I worked hard at banishing sexual thoughts of Rod from my mind. It just didn't seem right. Like I was committing adultery in my heart. But one afternoon, I found myself watching him from the window as he swam in his pool. After a while, he climbed out and lay back on a lounge chair on the pool deck. His wet suit clung to every curve of his genitalia, and I started picturing him nude again. Before I knew it, I was fantasizing myself in his arms, having sex with him on the lounge chair, in the pool, out of the pool, in the sun, in the rain, in my bed, in his bed, all the while stroking myself with my fingers until I had an explosive climax.

That night I was all over Monte. We had another great sexual experience. The next morning, I thought it over. Monte was having a good time. I was having a good time. Nobody knew what was going on in my head. What harm was it doing if I was fantasizing about sex with my neighbor Rod? None at all, that's what.

I guess Monte would feel threatened if he knew that whenever we have intercourse I'm imagining another man's penis entering me and another man's lips on me. But there's no reason in the world why I should tell him. Is there?

Remembered Threesome

$\mathcal{A}$t twenty-three, Harry is about five feet ten inches tall and a little on the thin side. His shoulders and arms are disproportionately strong from lifting and carrying heavy video equipment on his job as a TV camera operator. He has brown hair, brown eyes, and a sparse brown moustache. His easy temperament is an asset in the high-stress broadcast news business.

The station I work for likes to send me on out-of-town assignments because they know I can get along with just about anybody. Hey, life is too short to waste on tension and uptightness. The trick is to have fun.

I mostly cover sporting events. I like traveling, but I know it's kind of hard on my wife, Felicia. We've only been married a few months, and I've already been away on four assignments. I guess she knew what she was getting into when she asked me to marry her. Maybe, like they say, absence makes the heart grow fonder. When I get home we're usually both so hot for each other that the sparks really get to flying. Once, though, a few sparks flew while I was away. I'll tell you all about it.

Actually, it was my first trip out of town after we got married. Fooling around with other women was the last thing on my mind, honestly. I believe in marriage and I believe in being faithful. So when I dropped into that hotel bar, it was only for a drink, just because I was feeling kind of lonely in my room. I was covering a basketball series and was going to be out of town for two or three more days. I really was wishing I was home.

When I sat down on the bar stool and ordered a beer, I hardly noticed the two women sitting together a few seats away from me. By the time I ordered my second beer, they had moved to take seats on either side of me. One of them, a tall dark-haired woman with a slim, boyish figure, said, "Hi, there. I'm Robin." Indicating the other, a shorter, fleshy blonde, she added, "This is my friend Trina. Are you just passing through?"

I wasn't used to being approached by strange women in bars. To tell you the truth, I thought they might be hookers at first. By the fourth beer, I learned they had been to the basketball game that afternoon and had seen me slinging my camera. I figured they just wanted to talk about basketball and about TV. Seems like everybody is fascinated by television people. Even a cameraman is some kind of celebrity.

Anyway, we talked about lots of things, most of which I don't even remember. I was feeling a little buzzed from the beers and was just about to order a fifth one when Trina said, "I've got a better idea. Instead of sitting here getting wasted, why don't we all go up to your room and have a really hot time."

I wasn't sure I heard right. What did she mean by a hot time? Could she mean what I thought she meant? I couldn't really believe it. Then I started thinking maybe they were hookers again. I decided to play along, knowing that if they were, nothing would happen until I paid in advance. I had no intention of paying anybody for anything. So I said, "Okay, let's see what develops."

Arm in arm, the three of us walked, a little shaky, to the elevators and took one of them to the seventh floor. I opened the door to my room with that little plastic key they give you in the nicer places and stepped inside. The two women followed.

"You have a better room than ours," Robin said. I thought, Hmmm, if they're staying here, maybe they're not hookers. But then, what do they want with me?

Without a word, Trina began undoing her black patent-leather belt. In a moment, she had it off and tossed it on the floor. She was wearing a gray dress, kind of short. She quickly unbuttoned the front and peeled it off. Under it, she wore only a pair of silvery pantyhose. Nothing else. I could see her golden triangle through the nylon crotch.

She grabbed my hands and pressed them against her big, naked boobs. Her nipples were the color of pink bubble gum. I could see and feel them hardening to my touch. I couldn't believe what was happening. Evidently my cock did, because it stood straight up and said, Harry, make the most of this.

While I played with Trina's big tits, Robin began stroking my ass through my jeans. I could feel my cock jumping. She must have seen it. She started rubbing it until I thought I would wet my pants. Trina threw her arms around me and pulled me against her for a hot passionate kiss, all tongues, while Robin unbuttoned my pants and started slipping them down.

It's all kind of hazy in retrospect, but within a few minutes, all three of us were completely naked and heading for the bed. The two girls sort of wrestled me down so that I was lying on my back with my cock sticking straight up in the air. Then, both at the same time, they started licking it. I lifted my head and opened my eyes wide to watch what they were doing.

One mouth was at the base of my cock, the tongue licking little circles around the bottom of the shaft. The other was at the tip, taking me into her wet heat and rolling her tongue and lips all around the crown. I reached out to fill my hands with them.

I remember that Trina's tits were big, and heavy, and full, and made a real handful. Robin's were not much more than nipples, but these were big, and dark, and shaped like long brown cones, and very exciting to touch. The best part was feeling the difference between them, while both of them worked on my cock.

I felt fingertips caressing my nuts. While I watched, their tongues dueled, moving against each other as they slid over the skin of my hard-on. Robin reached out and put her hand on one of Trina's tits, rolling the nipple in her fingers while she kissed the other woman and licked my cock at the same time.

Soon, Trina's hands went to Robin's little titties, playing with her nipples and bringing sobs of pleasure from her. Both of them wrapped their lips around my cock at the base, moving upward together until they were kissing over the tip. Then they broke contact with me all together and began kissing and caressing each other. They had taken their mouths away from me just in time, because I was about to burst, and Lord knows, I wanted this to go on forever.

The two women kissing and touching each other's tits was about the most thrilling sight I had ever seen. Things started getting even hotter when Robin lay back and spread her legs. Trina got down between them and placed her face right next to Robin's pussy. There was a thick jungle of shiny black curls around it, but I could see the pink lips and purple clit very clearly as the blonde started to lick and slurp it.

As she ate out her friend, Trina lifted her shapely ass high into the air in an obvious invitation. I got down behind her and began licking her pussy from the rear, allowing my tongue to sweep up over her asshole every now and then. She wiggled her hips and worked harder at Robin's pussy, bringing more sobs of pleasure from the dark-haired girl.

Now Trina's pussy was coated with moisture, a combination of my saliva and the juices of her sex. I couldn't resist it any longer. Rising to my knees, I placed the tip of my cock at the door of her opening and drove myself inside with a single, long, deep, plunge. She reared back at me, helping to bury the entire length of my cock inside her, all the while continuing to suck on Robin's open puss.

I kept my eyes open the whole time so I could see my

cock sliding in and out of the blond woman and at the same time see her mouth working on the dark-haired one. I thought I had found a way of getting to heaven without dying. My body and brain were a blazing inferno, seething with an excitement I had never before experienced. Here were two women with nothing on their minds but sex, not just ordinary sex, but a level of sex that a person can wish for all life long and never get to experience. All they could think about was eating each other and fucking me.

We tried every position possible that night. I lay on my back fucking Robin while Trina got down between our legs and licked my cock as it slid in and out of her friend's pussy. The girls sixty-nined each other while I watched, grabbing whatever tits or ass or pussy happened to present itself. They got on their hands and knees next to each other and I slipped my cock in and out of one pussy, into the next, and back to the first.

I came whenever I felt like it, and so did they. As soon as I finished shooting the last of my cum, I'd get hard again and restart the whole process. Trina put my cock between her big tits while Robin squeezed them together around it. Robin worked my hard-on into her tight asshole while Trina licked her pussy. It was a night of sheer bliss.

At some point, when I was more satisfied than any man ever has a right to be, I fell asleep, with my hands on two different pussies at the same time. When I woke up, I was alone. I got dressed and went down to the lobby.

I walked around, hoping to run into the girls, but no luck. I even asked at the desk if there were any guests named Robin or Trina, but the clerk said he could only look up last names. Later, I watched for them at the game, but didn't see them. Afterwards, I asked the bartender if he knew anything about them. I drew another blank.

It was almost as if I was supposed to get just one night of heaven on earth, but no more than one. Hell, that's more than most men ever get to have, anyway. Even though I knew that, I sure wished I could get some more of it.

When the assignment was completed, I went home to Felicia. Of course, I can never tell her about it. Shoot, we were practically newlyweds. I couldn't let her know I'd already been unfaithful. Yet, somehow I feel that my sex life really won't be complete unless I get to do something like that again.

Since then, I've imagined a threesome with Felicia and Robin. I've imagined a threesome with Felicia and Trina. Sometimes, even all three of them, and me, of course. Other times, I imagine Felicia and me with other women; women I could see casually in the street, or women who are friends of ours. I'm tempted to tell Felicia about these fantasies, but I can never do that, either. She'd think she isn't enough for me because I don't love her enough. It kills me that the most exciting experience I ever had was with two complete strangers, and my wife, who I love more than anything, will never know anything about it.

FOUR
Watch Us

$\mathscr{T}$here is something contrary about human nature. We like to do what we're not supposed to do. Ever since Eve and Adam tasted that apple, most of us have found forbidden fruit to be the sweetest.

Sex and privacy are so closely tied together in our society's view that it is rare for anyone to be seen by others while having sex. Perhaps that is why hotels furnish their "lovers' suites" with mirrors on ceilings and walls. This enables guests to watch themselves, imagining how they would appear to a fantasy audience.

For some people, observing themselves making love is not enough. They want others to look at them, too. The thought that they will be seen adds a special spice to their erotic play. This chapter tells the stories of three such people.

Karl knows that the sex he has with his wife is visible to their best friends and he works at improving their view. On the other hand, "John" derives a thrill from knowing that strangers will see the goings-on in his marital bed, enhanced by the thought that the sights may stimulate the watchers to acts of self-gratification or mutual sexuality. Sondra remembers an exhibitionistic experience she had as a college student.

Although the three stories are quite different from one another, the people telling them all have one thing in common: Their desire to be on view is, and will remain, unspoken, at least as far as their spouses are concerned. There is something, however, perhaps the same urge that drives them to their sexual exhibitionism, that induces them to tell us.

Bedroom Mirror

*K*arl, thirty-one, is an automobile mechanic, employed in a shop that specializes in foreign cars. He is dark complected with a thick shock of curly black hair and an even thicker beard. His soft hazel eyes are all that prevent his appearance from being overpoweringly intense. He is of medium height with a powerful stocky build and the forward-leaning posture of a person with a compelling purpose. When he smiles, his white teeth flash.

I guess I'm pretty happy with where I am in life. Me and Maureen have been married for five years. Three years ago, we bought this brand-new house. Yeah, I know it's in a housing development, a tract, but that don't really bother us. The neighborhood is clean and pretty quiet. It's going to be a nice place for us to raise kids someday. For now, though, Maureen's got to work so we can pay for it.

We've got lots of great neighbors. Our best friends, Roger and Velma, live right next door to us. Me and Maureen get together with them most every weekend.

Roger and Velma are part of my secret, so let me tell you a little about them. They're about our age. Roger's a mechanic, like me. We don't work in the same shop, but close enough so that most days we carpool. Velma mostly stays home and takes care of their two kids. I know Maureen would like to spend more time with her, because she really likes Velma, but working don't leave much time for socializing.

Shit, work don't even leave much time for sex. But me and Maureen both have pretty sharp sexual appetites, so no matter how tired we both are at the end of a workday, we always manage to get in a little screwing. Maureen can be a real tiger in the sack. She likes to move around a lot and make lots of noise.

Our house is right next door to Roger and Velma's. They build them so close together in this tract, that sometimes my wife tries to stuff a pillow in her mouth so the neighbors won't hear her screaming when we're screwing and she's all riled up. We never realized that maybe they could see us. Not until one morning when Roger and I were driving in to work together.

After a few minutes in traffic, he cleared his throat a few times and said, "Er, Karl, I don't exactly know how to tell you this but . . ." I waited for him to finish what he was saying, but his voice just sort of trailed off.

Finally I said, "Tell me what?"

"Well," he began again, "I don't exactly know . . ."

"Ah, come on, cut the shit," I interrupted. "You said that already. Get to the fucking point, will you?"

"Well, okay," he said. "You know that mirror on the closet door in your bedroom?"

"Yeah," I answered, wondering what the hell he was talking about. "What of it?"

"Well," he continued, "when that closet door is open just a little bit, Velma and me can see you and Maureen reflected in it when you're in bed. Er, fucking."

I was confused. "Huh?" I asked. "Our window doesn't even face your bedroom. How can that be?"

"No," he answered. "We only see you from the den. Lately we've been watching you two instead of Jay Leno." He chuckled to himself for a minute, like he was remembering something he saw. "I guess I'm dumb for telling you this, because we've really been enjoying the show. But you're my friend, and I thought you ought to know."

"Why, you couple of Peeping Toms," I said, only half joking. "What exactly have you seen?"

"I don't think you want to know," he answered, with a snort.

"Fuck, yeah, I want to know," I insisted. "What exactly did you see?"

"We seen everything the two of you got and everything the two of you do," he answered. "Velma feels really guilty about it. But that don't stop her from admiring your cock. She says it's huge. Bigger than mine. Personally, I think she's full of shit."

I was a little stunned at the thought of my buddy's wife staring at my dick and comparing it to her hubby's. "Yeah? What else?" I insisted.

"Well," he began, "if you don't mind my saying so, your wife has a great pair of knockers. Man, those nipples. So big and so dark. I've seen you sucking on them and I'm filled with envy. You know Velma's got these little bitty titties, and I ain't complaining or nothing, but I can't help being a little jealous of those beauties of Maureen's. I've got a couple of peeks down the front of her blouse before, but nothing like seeing them fully exposed in that bedroom mirror."

He was starting to really warm up to the subject. "We don't need to rent no X-rated videos," he continued. "You guys put on one hell of a fuck show. Sometimes I wonder how you can screw so long without shooting your load. It just amazes me. Usually, by the time you're finished, Velma and I are so hot from watching that we fall on the floor and finish each other off in a matter of seconds. Whew, that's some hot stuff."

Suddenly, he seemed to remember the situation and got embarrassed. "Jesus," he said. "What the fuck am I saying? I guess I should be apologizing, huh?"

Somehow, though, the description he'd been giving me

was getting me hot. I could feel myself growing hard inside my work pants. "Tell me specifically about some of what you've seen," I asked. "Specifically."

This seemed to make him feel better about it all, and he went right back to his story. "Well," he said. "Like, last night. Maureen walks into the bedroom and you're right behind her. You sit down on the bed and she starts undressing for you, doing some kind of little sexy dance. We can see her unbutton her shirt and toss it over your head. We can see you squirming to get out from under it so you won't miss any of the show. Then we see her holding the cups of her pink bra, all filled with those giant tits of hers.

"She unhooks it and slips it off. Velma gasps, looking at those giant hooters. 'Hey, Rog,' she says to me. 'Would I turn you on more if I had big boobs like Maureen's?' Well you know a guy can only give one answer to a question like that. Fuck honesty. 'Hell no, babe,' I says. 'I just love the ones you got. I like them just fine.'

"At this point, Maureen is playing with her tits while you watch. I'm beginning to wonder if you're ever gonna get into the act. But then you get up and strip off all your clothes and the rest of hers. You pull her on top of you, and we watch the two of you rolling around on the bed together. A minute later, we know you're inside her by the way the two of you are moving. Only wish we could have seen the entry, but the mirror just didn't take us that far.

"Anyway, you guys just seemed to go on for fucking ever. Up and down. In and out. We couldn't hear you, but we could imagine the sounds you were both making. Finally, you settled down to a nice slow rhythm. Then I guess you both came, because you ended up lying side by side hugging and kissing."

"Jeez," I muttered. "I don't know what to say. I guess I'm glad you told me all this, but it's kind of embarrassing."

"Embarrassing for you?!" Roger said. "What should I say? I'm gonna tell you something else. Up until we found out we could watch you in that mirror, myself's and Velma's sex life seemed to be going to hell. I mean what with the kids and the job and the mortgage, and all that shit, we both kind of lost interest. But ever since we saw you two going at it, everything's changed. Like hardly a night goes by that we don't do it, too. Take it from me, it's great to be doing it again." Then his voice changed a little. "I guess that's all over now that the cat's out of the bag," he added, sounding a little sad.

"I don't know about that," I answered. I don't mind telling you, his story was really turning me on. I was wondering how it would have felt if I'd knew they were watching at the time it was happening. "Does Velma know you're telling me about this?"

"No," Roger answered. "I didn't know myself that I was going to tell you until I actually started. I think Velma would die of embarrassment if she thought you guys knew."

"Well, I think Maureen would die, too, if she knew what you've seen. So let's just keep it between yourself and myself. Okay?"

"Sure, Karl," Roger promised.

"I'm going to make a confession," I said. "I find it pretty exciting to know that you guys have been watching. As long as the girls don't know, I think I'd like to keep on the way things have been."

"What do you mean?" Roger asked.

"You guys be watching again tonight," I said. "And you'll see what I mean. Now tell me, how can I position that closet door to give you a better view?"

He said he thought it would improve things if I could open the closet door about eight inches or so more than usual. So when I got home that night, that's exactly what I did. By the time Maureen got there, everything was in place. We had dinner, watched a little TV, and then headed for bed, just like usual. I didn't want to do anything different to give it away. I sure was feeling different, though.

On the way into the bedroom, I whispered that I wanted to see her lay back and play with her pussy for a while. She does that for me sometimes, so it didn't seem out of line. I was real excited by the idea that tonight I wouldn't be the only one seeing it. Roger would be seeing it too. For some reason, I was even more excited by the idea that Velma would be seeing it. It was like I wanted them to know how sexy my wife is and how much she would do for me.

As I watched Maureen doing herself, I took my clothes off and stood over her with my cock right in her face. I wanted her to suck it. She got the message and took it into her mouth, her hands still working at her pussy. I closed my eyes and imagined Roger and Velma seeing my hard-on sliding in and watching my wife give me the world's greatest head. I was getting a bigger kick out of this than any blowjob I ever had in my life. It was incredible.

After a while, I got on the bed next to her and asked her to ride on my cock. I positioned myself so that her ass would be facing the mirror as she mounted me. I wanted to be sure they'd see my cock going into her pussy. When it went in, the thought of them watching made it feel ten times better than fucking ever did. I just couldn't believe it.

If Roger thought his sex life was improved by this, he should only know what it was doing for me. I was groaning when she started dragging her pussy up and down on my shaft. Usually, I can hold out a long time, but not that night. I came so fast that I think I shocked Maureen. She's not one to let an opportunity to come escape her, so she managed to go off just a few seconds after I did, filling the air with the music of her sexual cries.

Afterwards, we lay together cuddling, like we usually do. Even that was exciting, because I knew we had an audience. At that point, I almost blabbed the whole thing to Maureen. I mean if it made me feel so good, it seemed only right that I'd share that good feeling with her. Good thing a blast of reality stopped me.

If she knew, she'd freak out. She'd never be able to face Roger or Velma again, and she'd probably never talk to me, either. Oh, I guess eventually we'd make up and all, but I doubt that our sex life would ever fully recover.

So I decided to stick to my original plan not to tell her. That's the way it's been ever since. I still keep that closet door open to just the right angle and I still keep the window shades open. I still know that every time Maureen and I are making it the chances are our friends and neighbors are watching every move we make. I still perform for them a little and try to get Maureen into spots that will give them the maximum view. But I'm never going to tell her about it. Never! I mean, why fuck up a good thing?

College Party

*S*ondra, forty-one, is five feet six inches tall and has a soft fleshy body, which she prefers to describe as "voluptuous." Her thick hair is bleached a shade of blond that doesn't even pretend to be natural, but the effect against her oval brown eyes is dramatic and subtly erotic. There is something frank and open about her as she bares her life's secrets to strangers. She has been in the health-care industry ever since she got out of college.

I've always liked people. So it just seemed natural for me to get into a field where I could interact with lots of people and help them as much as possible. Even in school, I had a huge circle of friends. I always managed to get involved in their lives. Maybe that's why I never stayed with the same man for very long. Things always got too serious, too fast. As it is, I'm on my third marriage now and hope it's my last. But I can sincerely say I still love all the men I've ever been with.

In college, I had one boyfriend after another. Usually, his friends would become my friends, too. Then after we broke up, I'd keep the friends. When I got another boyfriend, I'd add a whole new group of friends, until, finally, I knew just about everybody on campus.

Those were wild days. We all drank and smoked dope and partied almost every night. It's amazing I managed to get good grades. In fact, it's amazing that I got through school at all. Oh, yes, things were so very loose. So very laid-back. I long for those days.

I remember one night going to a party with my guy of the moment, a boy named Kirk. I heard from him just a few months ago, too. He's living somewhere in the Midwest, with a wife and five kids. It's scary to think that could have been me. I'm still not ready for kids, even at my age. Fortunately, my present husband, Trent, feels the same way about it.

But, anyway, Kirk and I went to this party. I guess we were about twenty, like most of the other kids there. You could almost smell the hormones cooking in a room full of people that age. All anybody could think about was getting laid. Most of us lived in dorms where there wasn't a lot of privacy. So at these parties, we'd turn down the lights and fool around, all in one big room, with nobody much caring who else was around or what anybody else might see. I can remember lots of times the girls were half naked and the boys had their pants open and their young dicks showing. There was always plenty of wine and grass, so the atmosphere was ripe for young people to romance and explore their sexuality.

At this particular party everybody had a pretty good buzz on and the music was blasting on the record player—Jimi Hendrix, I think it was—when we all got down to the business of making out. Kirk and I had our tongues down each other's throats and our hands in each other's pants, as did most of the other kids in the room. I remember looking around and getting so aroused by the sights all around us. I guess part of the kick was knowing that they were seeing us, too, just like we were seeing them. As I look back on it, I think maybe those were the most exciting times in my life.

I guess I was a little drunker than I thought, because I started losing whatever inhibitions I had left. I tore open my shirt to expose my breasts to Kirk's mouth. Nobody wore a bra in those days. He started sucking hungrily on them while I moaned with pleasure. My eyes were almost closed, but I managed to look out through the slits to make sure somebody heard me and was watching. When I saw several pairs of eyes on us, I tugged at Kirk's pants until they were open and then I pulled out his cock. I started stroking it up and down, making it big and thick and hard. All the time, my eyes were wandering around the room, watching others do similar things, and most of all, watching them watch us. It was thrilling. To tell you the truth, I don't think the sex got me off as much as knowing that so many eyes were on us.

I had done stuff like that before, and the erotic kick it gave me was a familiar one. But, as I said, I was losing whatever inhibitions I had left, and something big was getting ready to happen. In all the time that we had been going to these parties, nobody actually fucked in front of the others. Lots of fooling around, nipple play, and cock action, but no real fucking. So in some compartment of my intoxicated mind, I decided it was time to be the first.

I pulled Kirk's shirt off, tossed it onto the couch next to mine, and grabbed him by the shoulders. For a moment, I considered climbing onto his lap and doing it right there. Then I thought, hey, why not really put on a show? I'll spread out and do it on the floor. I rolled backward and started to pull him down on top of me. As he crept up beside me on the floor, I lifted my hips and removed my pants. Now all I was wearing were flimsy pink panties, and I knew that anybody who looked would see that the crotch was good and wet. I mean I was hot.

While Kirk stripped off the rest of his clothing, I started moaning louder and louder, to be sure of gathering an audience. All the while, my eyes moved around the room. Some of the people had noticed us and were watching while they continued their own sex play. Others were so busy that they were not yet aware that we were bumping it up a notch.

Kirk was naked now, his strong young hard-on jutting out in front of him like a club. He reached for my panties and started to pull them off, but I grabbed his hands. "No," I murmured, loud enough to be heard by anybody who was listening. "Take them off with your teeth."

Kirk did as I instructed, taking the wet fabric in his teeth and pulling the panties slowly down over my hips while I lifted my ass high in the air. I saw more people noticing us and more eyes on us as the other couples indulged in their own little foreplay games. When the panties were down around my ankles, I kicked them off and spread my legs wide so that anybody looking could see my wet, open slit.

I'll never forget how excited it made me to think of myself being totally exposed to all those people. I could hear murmurs and moans in response to my demonstration. I imagined that some of the men were playing with their women while fantasizing about playing with me. It made me feel very, very sexy.

Kirk knelt between my legs. Holding his cock in his hand, he began rubbing its tip up and down the length of my slit, covering the throbbing head with my juice until it shined. I wanted him inside me. I wanted everyone to see him going inside me. So I said, almost at a shout, "Fuck me, Kirk. Fuck me now."

As his firm masculinity sank inside my pussy, I glanced around again, satisfied to notice that most of the people in the room had their eyes glued to us while they halfheartedly continued their making out. When the tip of his cock reached way back inside me, the pleasure became so intense that I forgot everyone else and closed my eyes to concentrate on the sensations. Our hips rocked together and apart. His dick slipped in and out, deeper with each stroke.

For a while I just lay there, absorbing the ecstasy of the moment. Then I heard a masculine voice say, "This is too good to keep in the dark." Through my eyelids, I was conscious of the lights being turned on. The moment I opened my eyes, I realized that we had become everybody's center of attention. All other sexplay had stopped. Everybody was just sitting there, some half undressed, observing Kirk and me fucking our way to paradise.

Of course, that made it even more pleasurable. I guess I started putting on a show for them. I think maybe Kirk was into the act also, because the both of us made more noise than we ever did before. Our movements became exaggerated and intensified. We screamed; we hollered; we yelled; we groaned. We rolled, and tossed, and bumped, and grinded, like a pair of epileptic Siamese twins joined at the groin and having an erotic seizure.

The fucking felt good, but I have to admit that the best part was knowing that all those people were watching us. That was really great; the epitome of erotic sensation! That night I discovered that exhibitionism is at the very core of my sexuality.

Looking back at it twenty years later, it seems like it went on forever, like we kept fucking for our audience until the sun came up. Probably that wasn't the way it happened at all. Young people tend to go off quickly, like cannons with hair triggers. At the time, though, we had no complaints. Neither did anyone else. When we were done, I was kind of hoping that some of the other couples in the room would follow our lead, but no one did.

Kirk and I stopped going out together soon afterward, so it never happened again. Somehow, after that, there just weren't any situations in which I could fuck while others watched. So I had to find other ways of exhibiting myself. Conventional ways, like bikinis on the beach, low-cut dresses. You know, the kind of exhibitionistic stuff that everybody does.

Eventually, I got married and started living a middle-class life. Now I'm on my third marriage and still living a middle-class life. Jeez, I wish I could tell my husband about the thrill of fucking in front of an audience. I truly wish he'd get into it with me. Even though I know my college days are over, I think we ought to be able to find some kind of situation in which we could do it.

But how the hell do you say something like that to an accountant? That's what my husband does for a living. Or to any other conventional guy, for that matter? Do I just say,

"Hey, you know, when I was in college I fucked this guy with a lot of people watching and I really enjoyed it. Wanna try it?" No way. It's just not something I can tell him about. So I guess it's going to have to be my secret memory.

Secret Videotape

The man who told us this story asked us to call him "John." He made us promise that we would give no physical description of him, except to say that he is in his early fifties and that he has an ordinary kind of job with access to a computer and nobody looking over his shoulder. He describes himself as a World Wide Web addict, saying he spends several hours a day surfing the Internet.

One of the great things about the Internet is I found out I'm not the only freak in the world. I'm telling you, there are so many different kinds of weirdos on the Web that I feel almost normal. All my life, I've thought of myself as some kind of a pervert and hid my true nature from everybody in the world. Even my wife. Hah!—especially my wife.

I don't know why. Maybe an analyst could tell me, but I don't really care. I've always gotten the strongest kick out of being seen naked by strangers. When I was a little kid, I took every opportunity to pull my pants down in public. Then, when I was a teenager, I used to find excuses to pee in the street, hoping some passing women would see me. As an adult, there have been three times when I was nearly arrested for exposing myself to women. I was lucky each time and finally realized I couldn't be lucky forever, so I gave it up.

I did such a good job of pretending to be like everybody else that I managed to find a good woman and get married. She has no idea whatsoever about the things that really turn me on. Almost as soon as we got married, I transferred my exhibitionistic desires to her. I would fantasize about people peeking at her while she got dressed, or undressed, or while she was using the bathroom. The best fantasies are about people watching us both while we make love.

We have a pretty good sex life. There would be plenty for somebody to see if they had a chance to watch us. Once, I suggested to my wife that we go to a swing club, not to have sex with other couples but just to watch them and let them watch us. She was absolutely mortified at the idea. No fucking way. What did I think she was? All that sort of crap.

Then, on the Internet, I found this spy shop that sells equipment, supposedly for industrial espionage. I bought a miniature video camera built into a fake smoke detector and installed it opposite our bed. The camera transmits images to a VCR in the next room. There are no wires or anything else to give it away.

I installed it one day while my wife was at work. I didn't tell her anything about it, of course. As soon as she got home, I dragged her into the bedroom for a quick fuck. Later, after she had gone to sleep, I played back the videotape. What a disappointment. The camera missed all the hot action. All I got was an occasional glimpse of her ass as we rolled around the bed.

I adjusted the camera the next day, and readjusted it the day after that. I ended up adjusting it about fifteen times before I got it aimed and focused just right. But then it was perfect. I could record an entire lovemaking session without her knowledge and play it back any time I wanted.

I'd seen a lot of ads on the Internet for swaps of home-made sex tapes. I guess my whole reason for getting the camera was so that I could get involved in them. When I got a real good tape of us I would make several copies so that I would have lots of videos to trade. I started answering ads and posted a few of my own, using one of those anonymous e-mail addresses that some companies offer for free.

Let me tell you, people worked out the most complicated

systems for swapping tapes while keeping their identities secret. I mean, P.O. boxes, forwarding addresses, all kinds of shit. One guy even asked me to leave a tape in a certain locker at the airport and hide the key under an ashtray next to a certain phone booth so he could pick it up later. I didn't do it, though. It was a little too James Bond for me.

The thing is that about half of these people turn out to be rip-offs. I mean, I would send them the tapes and get nothing in return. At first that pissed me off. But then, when I looked at the tapes I did receive, the ones from the people who weren't rip-offs, I found that I wasn't really interested in seeing them, anyway. I guess what turns me on isn't looking at others, but being seen by others. I think the fact that it's always strangers makes it even more exciting. I like to imagine how they're reacting to the tapes of me and my wife fucking, the shots of her tits and pussy, the shots of my cock. I'd really like it if some of them would write me, by e-mail, to tell me what they thought of the tapes I sent them, but nobody ever does. Anyhow, it's plenty exciting the way it is.

Now, every time I fuck my wife, I realize that somebody is going to end up seeing a tape of the whole session. Maybe they'll be jerking off to it, or maybe they'll be fucking while watching it. The idea really gets me hotter than hell. As a result, I screw my wife more often than I used to and I think I do a better job. Maybe knowing the camera is on us brings out the best in me.

Sometimes, I feel like telling her all about it, so that she can get the same kick that I do. But I know better. What turns me on doesn't necessarily turn her on. In fact, I know she'd be pissed. She might even kill me. It would certainly be the end of our marriage. So if you ever see one of my ads on the Internet, don't let anyone know who I am.

FIVE
Erotic Paraphernalia

*A*rtificial penises probably have been around as long as real ones. During the course of history, they have been fabricated from stone, wood, ivory, bone, steel, leather, and just about every other material imaginable. Sophocles mentioned their use in *Lysistrata*, which he wrote almost twenty-five hundred years ago. A story in the collection known as *One Thousand and One Arabian Nights*, and dating perhaps to the eighth century, suggested the use of a banana as a penis substitute.

Technology reaches into every aspect of modern life, so it should come as no surprise that modern dildos are made of space-age plastics and may be brought to vibrating life by tiny rechargeable batteries. Along with them, sex shops sell an abundance of other erotic toys, ranging from inflatable dolls with vibrating vulvas, mouths, and anuses to masturbation machines capable of use by six persons of mixed gender, all at the same time.

The people whose stories are told in this chapter have made the use of erotic paraphernalia a regular part of their sex lives. Libbey uses mechanical devices to supplement an otherwise unsatisfactory marriage. Chad, who is content with his relationship, has found a way to add special spice to it with one of the most highly advanced intercourse machines on the market. Like so many others, each has a reason for keeping unspoken the desires that lead to their interaction with erotic technology.

Sex Toys

*L*ibbey is what we'd call a young forty-three, with a slim, petite figure and quick, agile movements. If she stretches, she stands just at five feet two inches. She has big, green saucer eyes. Her short blond hair is cut and styled like that of figure skater Dorothy Hamill. She keeps herself in shape working out regularly at a gym, making it hard to believe that she's the mother of four grown children. There is something behind her broad smile, however, that suggests disappointment lurking at the core.

My husband, Marshall, is almost fifteen years older than I am. I was only eighteen when we got married, and he was already a captain. Now he's a lieutenant colonel. I don't think I'd better say any more than that, because if anyone in the army ever figured out who was telling you this, that would be about as far as he could ever expect to go. There's something about the military that tends to be a little narrow-minded.

Actually, that's the major problem in my marriage. My husband is a very strong-willed person. He's got to win every argument. Whenever there is a decision to be made, his word is always final. It was all right when I was eighteen and maybe even into my twenties, because I was just a kid then, and he was kind of like a father figure to me. But as I got older, it got more and more difficult for me. I knew I never really had a choice about it, so I just learned to accept it.

Our kids have had the same problem. They tell me I'm the

mellowest person they know and ask me why I don't fight for my rights with their dad. But I realize that would be pointless, so why get myself hurt banging my head against a stone wall?

All in all, life is okay. We've moved around quite a bit, but we've always lived in a nice place. We've traveled all over the world. We've never had money hardships, like so many other people do these days. That's how I rationalize my life.

Our love life has never been what you'd call great. Somehow, Marshall got the idea that the manly way to have sex is to shove it in, pump a couple of times, withdraw, and go right to sleep. Like taking a hill in southeast Asia, or something. Rush in, get what you come for, then get the hell out of there.

At first I didn't know any better. You might say I had a strict upbringing. My mother found ways of teaching me that sex was just for men. Decent women didn't really enjoy it. We just did it so we could have children, which is what we were made for. So in the middle of the night, when Marshall rolled me over and climbed on top of me, I did my duty and accepted it. Our four wonderful children were my rewards.

As I got older, I started to feel some kind of void within me. An emptiness that I just couldn't explain and didn't understand. I tried talking to other officers' wives, but I didn't even know how to describe what I was feeling. Even still, I got the distinct impression that many of them felt the same way, too.

Then, when we were stationed in Hawaii, I met Millie. She was a great gal. Lots of fun. Always laughing and joking around. One day we were drinking mai tais, and maybe Millie had a few too many, because she looked deep into my eyes and said, "You know, Libbey, I don't think you're getting laid enough." None of the ladies I knew used that kind of language, so I was a little taken aback. Before I had a chance to react, she added, "Well, if you want good sex you won't get it from an officer, that's for sure." When she stopped to take another sip of her drink, I decided to leave the subject alone. I felt relieved when she started talking about something else.

Afterwards, though, I couldn't help thinking about what she had said. About not getting laid enough and about not getting good sex from an officer. I wondered what she meant by all that. The next time we saw each other, I just came out and asked her. I was afraid she wouldn't even remember saying those things, but I was wrong.

"I guess I shot my mouth off," she said. "But every word of it is true. You can't expect to be happy, healthy, and wise if you aren't getting quality sex. I think the higher the rank of the officer, the less good sex his wife ever gets." Then in a lowered voice, she said, "I'll take an enlisted man, every time."

I was embarrassed. Millie was married to a full colonel. Was she telling me that she had affairs with enlisted men? My God, in the old days, they'd have drawn and quartered her for that. She might have been reading my mind because she laughed, moved closer to me, put her arm around my shoulders, and said, "Look, honey. You either find yourself a good strong lover or go out and buy a vibrator. If you don't get off, you'll go positively nuts!"

I had a vague idea of what she meant by getting off. I knew it was something I'd never experienced. Even if my mother was right, even if it was something decent women didn't do, I knew I'd always wanted it. But I certainly wasn't going to start cheating on my husband. I could never do anything like that.

I wanted to ask her what she meant about a vibrator, but, really, I already knew. After all, I'm an officer's wife, not a nun. I've seen ads in magazines and pretended to myself that I was shocked, when inside I knew I was actually fascinated. I've heard the double entendres on TV sitcoms. I knew what a vibrator was for. I was just too naive to realize that such things were designed for women like me. I didn't even know how I could go about getting one.

Millie read my mind again. "There are a few sex shops in the neighborhood, but they're all crawling with guys from the base. I know one on the other side of the island, where nobody ever goes. I've been there a few times and I've never seen anyone from around here. You can find all the paraphernalia you want there. I'd offer to take you, but I have a feeling you'd rather do this alone." Although I tried to act as though I wasn't interested, I paid very close attention as Millie gave me the name of the shop and directions for finding it.

The next day I drove there. I don't know what I expected, but this place certainly wasn't it. It was clean and airy and not the least bit sleazy. To my surprise, there was a woman sitting behind the counter. When I walked in, I was a little dazed by the open displays of sexual items. For a moment, I just stood there staring. "Can I help you?" she asked, like a clerk in any other retail store would have.

"Thanks," I said. "I think I'll just look around." As I strolled through the shop, I couldn't believe the things I was seeing. There were racks and racks of adult videos. There were artificial penises and long tapering vibrators. Their use was obvious enough. There were also inflatable dolls, silver balls, clamps of all kinds, big plastic balls strung together like pearls, board games, decks of playing cards, even computer software. I couldn't even figure out what half of the stuff was for.

Then I saw a box marked "Do-It-Yourself Do-It-Yourself Kit," priced at $49.95. The label said, "Complete Instructions for Use Included." I thought this was just the right product for a beginner like me, so, with some trepidation, I picked it up and carried it to the counter. The woman took it from me without a word and rang up the purchase on the cash register. Then she told me the price, with tax, and placed my purchase in a brown paper bag. Naturally, I paid cash. How would I ever explain a check written to a place like this?

I rushed home, but Marshall was already there when I arrived, so I had to carry my purchase into the bedroom and hide it in one of the drawers of my dresser. After dinner, we watched TV for a while and then went to bed. I was just about to fall asleep when Marshall climbed on top of me for one of his quickies. I let him do what he wanted, wondering all the while how I would use the sex toys I had bought. It was over in less than a minute.

I was still asleep when Marshall left the following morning. My very first thought was about the do-it-yourself kit buried under my sweaters. I was dying to look at it and read the instructions in the box. In my nightgown, I got it from the drawer and brought it to the bed.

With nervous fingers, I opened the box. Inside were three items: a long plastic vibrator, an artificial penis made of pink rubber and covered with little bumps, and a string of plastic balls. There were also two batteries, shrink-wrapped in plastic. The "instructions" said only that batteries should be inserted in the vibrator, leaving it to me to figure out what to do next. There was also a little slip of paper that said that in Asian cultures the plastic balls are inserted into the female organ and pulled out, one at a time, at the moment of orgasm.

I decided to try the vibrator first, because that was what Millie had recommended. I unwrapped the batteries and put them into the device, all the while feeling as though I were being watched. I remember that I kept looking around the room in paranoia. Finally, the batteries were in, the cap was screwed back on the vibrator, and I was ready to begin. But what was I supposed to do next?

I lay back on the bed and pulled my nightgown up over my hips. There was something very naughty about exposing my vagina that way, even though there was no one there to see it. I can't ever remember Marshall ever taking the trouble to look at me down there.

I reached down and touched myself with my hand, noticing how dry I felt. I thought it would be hard to get that plastic tube inside me, but I just had to try. So I flipped the little switch at its base. When it started vibrating, I placed it at the opening of my vulva and began pushing it in.

At first it hurt a little, because I was so dry and because I guess my body just naturally rejected this unnatural intrusion. But after a couple of moments, my body began to receive it. I was becoming moist and my tissues were sort of flowering open. I pushed it in slowly, trying to treat myself with all the tenderness that I was lacking from Marshall.

I had it in maybe four or five inches when the vibrations started feeling uncomfortable. It tickled, sort of. So I started drawing it out. When I did, my hand moved accidentally upward. Without meaning to do so, I ended up dragging the shaft of the vibrator along the top of my slit, against that little bump there that I had barely been aware of before.

I knew it would swell sometimes. When it did it would kind of itch, but I never associated it with feelings of pleasure. Yet now that the plastic device was vibrating against it, I was experiencing pleasure that was absolutely intense.

I had found a magic spot. It felt deliciously warm and sensual. It must be the clitoris. I had heard of it, but always thought there was a controversy about whether it really existed. Now I knew. It existed all right. Did it ever!

I pulled the vibrator all the way out of my vagina and placed its tip right against the spot. The closer I got to the middle of it, the better it felt. Within seconds, that little spot grew larger and larger, until my whole body seemed to be revolving around it. By now I was wetter than I'd ever been.

I could feel moisture all over the insides of my thighs and matting the hair around my vulva. Sometimes after Marshall was finished with me, I'd be wet there, too, from his ejaculation. But this was different. This moisture was all from me.

I had never felt such wonderful pleasure in all my life. I got more and more tingly, first just around the clitoris, and then running all through my body. I writhed on the bed, grinding my bottom against the mattress.

My breath was coming in deep, heavy drafts. My heart was beating faster and faster. I felt chills rushing over me, making me shudder uncontrollably. I was convulsed with feelings I never knew before.

Suddenly, I was filled with fear. Something horrible was building. I was going to blow apart. I was going to lose my mind. I was losing all contact with the world. Then it happened.

I'll never forget how it felt when that first orgasm hit me. It was like an eruption inside that had been waiting far too long to let loose. It shattered all my bones and made my head spin crazily. I must have been making animal noises, because I felt like a rutting beast. It was just too good. I wasn't going to be able to stand it anymore.

I had to stop the vibrator. But I couldn't. I had to stop. I had to go on. I wanted it to end. I wanted more. And more. And more. I heard myself scream. Then I sort of passed out.

I didn't really lose consciousness. I just lost control over my body. The hand holding the vibrator fell to my side and lay on the bed, like a bird that had flown into a pane of glass. The vibrator kept buzzing, but I didn't even hear it. Eventually, I slipped into a weird sleep, filled with dreams of men with huge penises lining up to take me one after another. When I woke up, I was more rested than I had ever been.

That morning was a turning point in my marriage and in my life. All the frustration that had been bottled up inside me and that I had been feeling without even knowing it was gone. Relief was just a vibrator away. Everything got better. The sun even seemed to be brighter. Now, instead of feeling disappointment, I could concentrate on the good things in my life. When I needed satisfaction, I could give it to myself.

I've been back to that little sex shop many times since that day. I've bought just about every sex toy they have: nipple clamps, ben-wa balls, velvet manacles, feathers, butt plugs. I've even gotten up the nerve to ask the woman who works there for recommendations. Some of the things I bought turned out to be too weird or just not pleasurable. But others have enhanced my newfound sexuality.

I haven't told Marshall about any of this, of course. Nothing will ever change him, so what would be the point of telling him something that would only make him feel threatened or convince him that I'm some kind of sex freak? I wish things could be different and I could somehow make him understand that I have needs just as real as his. But for now I'll just have to settle for the way things are.

Sybian

*C*had is a weekend surfer and looks it, with longish, sun-bleached hair and sparkling blue eyes. His skin is tan and his body is lean. At twenty-five, he has a strong but boyish appearance, standing about six feet tall, with broad shoulders and muscular thighs that show below the frayed bottoms of the cut-off jeans he is wearing when we meet him. He always seems to be smiling, as though just being alive is a pleasure. It's hard to picture him wearing a suit when he goes to work at the large insurance of office where he is employed.

Hey, everybody's gotta eat, and that means you gotta have a job. If you got any brains, though, you keep everything in perspective. Work is work, and play is play. Nobody should work any more than they have to. The rest of the time is for living and having fun. My job worked out to be a source of fun, too. But don't let me get ahead of myself.

I got a great girlfriend. We've been living together for a little more than a year. As far as I'm concerned, it's permanent. She likes the same things I do—surfing on the weekends, and lots of good, hot sex. Nothing turns me on more than seeing her get off. I'll do anything to make her come. I love to eat her pussy for hours on end. I wish I could fuck as long as that, but I tend to pop kind of quick. That's why I got her this gizmo.

It's called a Sybian and it's the most incredible fucking machine ever invented. When I saw a promotional video showing what it could do, I knew I just had to buy it for her, even though it cost more than two weeks' salary. Fourteen hundred bucks, to be exact. I'll tell you this, though, it's been worth every nickel.

I gave it to Emma for Valentine's Day, all wrapped up in tissue paper with hearts on it and a big red bow. When she opened the package, I could see she had no idea what it was. The thing is shaped like a small barrel, cut down the middle the long way. It's covered in brown vinyl and has a little plastic rod sticking up from the center of its rounded top. There's a cable connected to it with a control box at the end, containing a series of dials. Emma just sat there looking at it, with a question mark on her face.

I opened the box of accessories that came with it and took out one of the inserts. When she saw it, I could see understanding beginning to dawn in her eyes. The insert is shaped like a cock, made of soft plastic with a texture like skin. It's got ridges all around it and is connected to a plastic flap with little knobs sticking up. There were two more like it in the box, each a different size. Also one shaped like a long pointing finger.

I took the medium-sized cock-shaped one and fitted it onto the plastic rod. Now the thing looked like a gymnast's vaulting horse in miniature with this plastic dildo sticking out of it. I picked up the control box and started fooling with the dials.

One of them made the dildo vibrate, regulating the speed from very, very slow to incredibly fast. Another made it pump up and down, just like a real cock would do inside a woman's pussy. It also had a speed control so it could fuck as slow or as fast as anyone might want. The third dial made the plastic prick rotate, kind of like a finger pointing up and making little circles in the air.

Emma just couldn't believe that anyone had taken the trouble to invent such a complex fucking machine. I could see that she was dying to try it, and I was real eager to see it in action. So I said, "Go ahead, baby. I want to watch you get fucked by it."

She was in such a hurry that she didn't even bother to take all her clothes off. She just dropped her pants, peeled off her panties, and squatted down over the thing. Before she settled onto the dildo, I rubbed some lubricant on it, like the booklet that came with it recommended. Then I watched as she lowered herself down and her pussy swallowed the plastic cock.

When it was all the way inside her, I handed her the control box and sat back to watch the show. She started playing with the dials, one at a time. Each time she made a little adjustment, I could see the expression on her face changing. Her pussy got all frothy and foamy as her juices started flowing. I couldn't see what was going on inside, but I could imagine it.

Within seconds, she started moaning and groaning in that way I recognized. It was incredible, but she was coming already. Sometimes when we fucked, it would take her fifteen minutes of good solid thrusting before she got off. That Sybian machine got to her so fast I just couldn't believe it.

I thought it was over and was sorry it had ended so fast. Boy, was I mistaken. It hadn't ended at all. The second she finished coming, I could see her getting all turned on again. Like she was going from one orgasm to the next without even stopping for breath. She was panting like a bitch in heat, moaning stuff like, "Oh, God, this feels so good. Oh, I can't believe it. Oh, I'm going to come again. Oh no, oh yes, oh God, oh here I come." Unbelievably, her second climax was beginning just a few minutes after the first one ended.

After that she still wasn't finished. With her eyes closed tightly, she just let the control box slip from her hands and gave herself over completely to the sensations the Sybian was delivering. I picked up the box and started fooling with it, turning the vibration dial both ways to make it go faster and then slower.

By her reaction, I could see what speed she liked best, so I played with it, bringing her up and down with ease. I started doing the same with the other two dials, raising her up to the level of climax and then easing her back away from it. Up and down. Up and down. This time, when she came, I felt responsible for it. I was controlling the sensations and doing everything I possibly could to make it great for her.

We played with the machine for a couple of hours. She never got tired of it. She just rode it to glory again and again. I never knew any woman was capable of so many orgasms. There didn't seem to be any end to the pleasure she could take from it.

My cock was so hard from watching that I took off my pants and started rubbing it. I was about to shoot my load, when she got off the machine, pushed me back on the floor and mounted me, burying my hard-on in her pussy and riding me the way she had been riding the Sybian. I came within seconds, filling her with hot gism. Miraculously, she came again, this time with me.

When I was done, I sighed deeply and lay back in a state of total relaxation. She lay next to me and rubbed up against me. "Oh, thank you, baby," she whispered. "That's the best present I ever got. I think we're both going to have more fun with it than we ever imagined two people could."

After a rest, she got on the Sybian again and got herself off a couple more times. I just played with my cock until I came from watching her. It was fun to see how excited she got and to let my cum fly as I stroked myself to climax. That night we slept like babies. When morning came, she got on the machine again before taking her shower and getting dressed for work.

I was so glad I bought it for her that I just had to tell someone about it. That morning, at the office, while I was in the coffee room with one of the other guys, I started talking about the wonderful fuck machine I had bought my girl for Valentine's Day. He just snickered, one of those dirty little laughs that made me feel guilty for telling him private stuff about Emma.

Doris, a secretary I had seen around but barely knew, was in the coffee room and overheard. The minute the jerk left, she came to me and admitted that she had been eavesdropping. She asked me to tell her all about the machine.

I started describing it to her. First, just the device itself, how it was shaped, how it worked, stuff like that. Then I talked about how much it had turned my girlfriend on to use it and how excited it made me to watch her. Doris was enthralled.

"Wow," she said. "Ever since I broke up with my boyfriend, I've been feeling sexually frustrated. Sometimes, I think of going out to one of those singles bars just to pick up a guy for sex, but that's so dangerous these days. Maybe that Sybian is the answer to all my problems. Can I ask how much it cost?"

When I told her, her face fell. "Oh, God," she said. "It's probably worth it, but I could never afford that. I can barely pay my rent, as it is. I sure wish I could try one, though."

I don't really know what possessed me to say it, but I blurted out, "Well, maybe you can try Emma's."

Doris's eyes sparkled. "Oh," she said. "Could I?"

"Yes," I said a little hesitantly. "On two conditions. First, it's gotta be our secret. Emma wouldn't like it at all if she knew about it."

"That's no problem for me," Doris said. "I wouldn't want anyone to know either. What's the second condition?"

I swallowed hard before answering her. "I get to watch," I said. "Just watch. I promise I won't try anything with you."

She looked at me coldly for a long minute, and I started thinking about sexual harassment. Shit, what had I done? Maybe I should just try to laugh it off and say I was only joking. Then she surprised me. "Okay," she said. "It's a deal. But all you do is watch. Agreed?"

I was so excited that I was too out of breath to answer at first. Finally, I swallowed again and said, "Agreed."

Emma's and my apartment is only a few blocks from the office where I work. So I asked Doris if she'd like to try it that very afternoon at lunchtime. She said yes. I told her to meet me in the office lobby at twelve o'clock. When the time came, I was shaking like a leaf.

We left the building and hurried to the apartment. I was so turned on by the thought of what was happening that I felt like running all the way. But somehow I managed to maintain. I could see that Doris was nervous, too. I don't know whether it was because she'd be doing it in front of me or just because she was excited about trying the Sybian.

When we got into the apartment, I led her straight to the bedroom. The Sybian was still set up on the floor where Emma and I had left it. There were some condoms in my night table drawer, and I put one on the plastic dildo before covering it with lubricant. "There it is," I said. "Have a ball."

Doris stood there for a minute looking at the machine and licking her lips. Then she reached under her skirt and removed her panties, rolling them down her legs and kicking them off. She lifted her wide skirt to the waist, giving me a little glimpse of the dark hair that surrounded her pussy as she squatted down over the Sybian and eased the dildo inside her. "What do I do now?" she asked.

I picked up the control box and showed it to her. "This one works the vibrator," I said, giving the dial a little twist. As soon as I did, I saw her body jump and I knew the little plastic cock was doing its work inside her. "This one controls the thrust," I added, turning dial number two. She made a gurgling sound as the device started to fuck her. "And this one," I said, turning the final dial, "makes it go round and round inside."

I could see that my explanation was unnecessary. She already knew what the machine was capable of doing. Her sobs and moans were telling me that. She started to ride it, as if it was a bronco at the rodeo, issuing little cries of pleasure. She didn't seem the least bit embarrassed. In fact, she hardly seemed aware that I was in the room.

There was something so sexy about having this woman I barely knew in my bedroom fucking herself with Emma's new toy. It went straight to my cock, which was so hard that it ached. If she looked, she would have seen it pressing against the front of my pants, where it left a little spot of moisture. But she was much too busy to see anything besides the pretty pictures in her head.

Even though I didn't know her, I could tell that she was about to come. The way her head was moving, the way her hips were bucking, the way her throat was tightening, all made it so obvious that she might as well have shouted it to the world. Even after she came, she wouldn't quit, riding the perpetual fucking machine to another orgasm and then another.

If we didn't both have to get back to work, I think she would have stayed there fucking herself with the machine until Emma came home and caught us. After a while, I had to stop her and tell her what time it was getting to be. When she shut off the controls, she didn't look the least bit disappointed. In fact, her face was wearing an expression of total satisfaction.

"Oh, God, Chad," she said. "This was great. I don't know how to thank you. Do you think I can do it again sometime?"

Was she kidding? It was about the most erotic thing I ever saw. You're goddam right she could do it again. All I said was, "Sure, I guess so. As long as no one finds out."

She was quiet for a minute as she put her panties back on. Then she said, "Do you think I can just tell one person about it? My best friend, Alice. I just know she'd want to hear about this."

"I don't know," I said, a little nervous. "I wouldn't want word to start getting around the office."

"Don't worry," Doris answered. "She doesn't work with us. She works in a department store down the street. Do you think you might be willing to let her try it sometime?"

That did it. Of course I'd be willing. I couldn't wait to see another woman riding Emma's Sybian. This was turning out to be the best investment I ever made.

Alice called me the next day and said that her friend Doris had told her all about it. We made a date to meet at lunchtime on the corner by my apartment building. She was a real beauty—Latin, with huge tits and big black eyes. When I brought her into the bedroom, she took off all her clothes and rode the Sybian totally naked. It was quite a sight.

A few days later, I got a call from a friend of Alice's, who also wanted to try the gizmo. After that, there seemed to be a steady stream of women who were willing to let me watch in return for a chance at the world's greatest fucking machine. Some acted a little shy, keeping as much of their clothing on as possible. Others were totally uninhibited, letting me get a good look at their tits and pussy as they rode the Sybian to climax after climax. Either way, I get fantastically turned on seeing them get off on the device.

All I ever do is watch. That's enough for me, because it gets me so hot that afterwards all I can think of is making love to Emma. We fuck like mad every night, between her sessions on the Sybian. I find that I can last longer and longer and sometimes I can even get her off two or three times in a row myself. Naturally, I'm thinking all the while of the different women I've seen riding her machine.

Will I ever tell her? I don't see how I can. First of all, she wouldn't like the idea of anyone else using her intimate machine, even though I always cover the dildo with a condom. Second of all, I know she sure as hell wouldn't like thinking of me in our bedroom with all those naked women, watching them come again and again. I don't think she'd believe that all I ever do is watch. Even if she did believe it, I don't think she'd tolerate it. Anyway, there isn't any particular reason why I should tell her. Some things are best left unspoken, aren't they?

SIX
Sexual Slavery

*H*umans are equipped with many inhibitions about sex. Some experts have suggested that these inhibitions originally came into being to protect the social structures we developed before evolving to our present state. Among apes, for example, if a female is caught by her usual mate in the act of copulating with a different male, she may scream and fight and pretend that she was being taken against her will. Apparently, this relieves her of the social guilt connected with her offense and brings forgiveness from the alpha ape.

Perhaps this explains why stories of sexual slavery are common in pornography. Our research shows that many people imagine being forced against their wills to serve the sexual needs of others. Some actually arrange to have such experiences. This permits them to indulge their own erotic appetites without taking responsibility for violating the moral codes established by society.

For one of the people whose stories are told in this chapter, sexual slavery exists only in her imagination, a delightful masturbation fantasy that amuses her but does not involve her in any forbidden activity. Another imposes a form of slavery on himself, by pretending to take seriously an obligation that he could easily have shrugged off. Although true slavery is rare in modern society, the third story is about a man who was an actual sex slave, while forced to share a prison cell with a monster known as Big Jim.

Each of the people who told us these stories admitted, in one way or another, that there was something pleasurable about being forced to satisfy another's sexual needs. None, however, was willing to admit this to a life-partner, or even to acknowledge that the fantasy or experience of being a sex slave had occurred. For all, the idea of being erotically used and abused against their wills remains, and ever will remain, an unspoken desire.

Auction

*A*rtie, forty-two, is in construction. He says he does whatever jobs comes along, but prefers steel work. He is five feet nine or ten inches tall, with powerful, beefy shoulders and a barrel chest. Even when sitting still, his well-toned muscles are flexed, demonstrating his strength. His hair is short and the color of butterscotch. His eyes are brown. He wears a good-natured smile and has an uninhibited manner of talking.

Yeah, I've got a sex secret. It's a hot one. I spend lots of time thinking about it, remembering that great afternoon.

I've been a member of the Stags Society for a very long time. It's one of those benevolent organizations, you know. Do stuff for the community and all that. My reason for joining, and probably most of the other guys too, was just to be able to get away from the wife one night a week. We have these business meetings, where we plan events and things. After that, we play cards.

Every year we have a big fund-raising event. The money goes to some deserving high school senior, as a scholarship to help pay his way through college. It's a worthy cause, but I think we all do it mainly for the fun. We ask the local merchants to donate stuff. Most of the members kick in something, too. Then we sell it at auction.

Two years ago, I donated six hours of slave time. That's what people give when they don't have any real stuff to contribute. Usually, the high bidder has a fence they want painted or some windows they want washed. I figured I'd spend a Saturday afternoon doing my good deed to help some kid go to school. Like buying a ticket to heaven, if you know what I mean. Well, anyways, it turned out to be a ticket to heaven on earth.

At the auction, when it came time to sell my contribution, Mac—he's the auctioneer—had me stand up on stage and turn around three hundred and sixty degrees. "Look at this strapping worker," he said to the crowd. "Six hours of slave time can be yours. What am I bid? What am I bid?" Mac is pretty good at it. He managed to get the bidding up to a hundred and ten bucks for the cause.

The winner was a girl in her twenties. When it came time to settle up, she introduced herself to me and said her and her partners needed their house cleaned. I was expecting some kind of work a little heavier than that, but what the hell, a slave is a slave. So I said, Okay, I'd be there that weekend.

When I showed up, they turned out to be three girls sharing a house. It really was a mess, looked like a war zone. I figured I'd have my six hours cut out for me. "Where do you want me to start?" I asked.

"To begin with," one of them said. "You did agree to be our slave. So we want you to call each of us 'Mistress.' "

I was a little taken aback, but what the hell, I'd go along with the fun. "Yes, Mistress," I said, putting on a grin.

Another one piped up. "You'll have to work nude," she said. "Slaves do as they're told."

"What the fu—er, what the hell are you talking about?" I sputtered. "I'm here to clean your house."

"Not exactly," the third one answered. "You're here to be our slave for six hours. That's what we bought and that's what we paid for. Now get those clothes off, slave."

I gotta be honest with you, the idea was beginning to appeal to me a little. I mean, these were pretty good-looking girls and they were maybe fifteen years younger than me. It was flattering that they wanted to see me in the buff. "Yes,

Mistress," I said, starting to enjoy this. "Where can I go to get undressed?"

"Right here," the first one said. "And be quick about it, slave."

Oooh, I liked that. So I do what I'm told. In front of those three pairs of eyes, I reach for the buckle of my belt and start tugging at it. I gotta tell you, I found it awful hard to look at those gals while I was getting out of my clothes. Pretty much, I stared at the floor. Next thing you know, I was naked. My cock was starting to stir, too. Not a full hard-on, if you know what I mean, but kind of a semi-hard.

When I was done, I looked around and saw that they were all watching me, mostly staring at my cock. That made it a little stiffer. I was really embarrassed. One of them handed me a feather duster and said, "Okay, now, slave, get to work. You can start right here in the living room."

I felt foolish standing there stark-naked with this silly little feather duster in my hand, but a slave is a slave. So I started making swipes at the tabletops and stuff with the feathers, trying to forget that I was stark-naked. Pretty soon, I heard the girls leaving the room and I figured I was alone. That was a relief.

Then I heard someone clearing their throat. I guess I wasn't alone after all. I looked up, and there was this one girl on the couch. She had her skirt pulled up around her waist. One leg was thrown over the arm of the couch and her other foot was on the floor. She had no panties on. I had a good, clear view of her pussy, which was spread wide. I just stared at it, not knowing what to do or say.

"Come here, slave," she commanded. "I want you to eat me."

I didn't exactly know what kind of game she was playing, but I was perfectly willing to play it too. I dropped to my knees before her and, like a good, obedient slave, went to work on her pussy. But first I said, "Yes, Mistress."

I licked and sucked, burying my face in that young quim until she was flowing like a fountain. Her voice grunted with pleasure. I kept eating her out until she was finished coming. After a couple of seconds, she sighed and said, "Okay, you can go back to your duties now." I wasn't sure what she meant until she added, "Dust, slave."

So I started swinging that stupid little feather duster again. I heard her leave the room and figured my sexual job was done. But no sooner was she gone than another girl came into the room. This one was as naked as I was. She stood at the end of the coffee table and bent over it, putting her hands on its surface. "Slave," she ordered, "come here and fuck me."

I was ready to obey that command, all right. "Yes, Mistress," I said, dropping the duster and walking over to stand behind her. My cock was as hard as a rock and jumping all over the place. I used my hands to spread the cheeks of her ass and expose her drooling pussy. Then I slipped it right in. I started humping in and out when I heard the third girl enter the room. I looked up and saw her. She was naked, too.

"Go ahead. Don't let me stop you," she said. "I want to watch." She added, "You better not come, slave. Because I'm next." She stood there breathing hard while I fucked her friend.

I'm pretty good at holding back, so I didn't have any problem at all keeping it up until the little sweetie came. She let out a series of shrill gasps and cries that sounded like a whole nest of birdies. When I pulled my cock out of her, it was dripping wet with the juices of her twat.

The other girl was already lying on the floor. Her legs were spread, and she was pointing to her pussy with one finger of each hand. "Put it right here," she said.

I liked the idea of fucking her while my prick was coated with the other one's juice. "Oh, yes, Mistress," I said, as I fell to the floor between her thighs. I stuck my cock right in.

Just as I felt her pussy closing around it, she commanded, "Don't come in me, slave. I'm off the pill."

While I fucked her, the other two girls stood and stared. That made it even hotter. I pounded for a good long time until she finished coming. Then, obeying her order, I pulled out and let my own stuff shoot all over her naked belly. The other two applauded like it was an opera performance or something.

When I was done, one of them said, "You still owe us five hours of slave time. You can finish cleaning the house." Which is what I did. Naturally, as far as my wife knows, cleaning the house was all I did.

The following year, I donated six hours of slave time to the auction again. Unfortunately for me, the high bidder was an elderly couple who needed their attic cleaned out and their trash hauled. I'm going to give it one more shot, but I don't suppose I'll ever get lucky again, like I did that first time.

Meanwhile, I think about those three girls constantly. I liked the way they called me "slave" and ordered me around. I even liked calling them "Mistress." It made the fucking more exciting. Sometimes, when I'm screwing my wife, I close my eyes and remember that glorious afternoon when I was a sex slave to three young women, one right after another.

Poker Slut

$\mathcal{A}$t twenty-six, Cynthia is an architect, struggling up the ladder on the partnership track at a large firm. Although she dresses in severe, dark suits, they do little to disguise her femininity, which perhaps is better described as a kind of raw sexuality. It radiates from her flashing blue eyes and heart-shaped face. She shows it in every toss of her wavy black hair. Her figure is the classic hourglass, with sensuously rounded breasts and a narrow waist. She is tall and soft, with a warm and disarming smile.

Brady is four years older than I am, and we have a very satisfying sex life. We've only been married two years, after living together for one, but in that short time we've fully explored each other's sexuality. Well, almost fully. There's one little fantasy I've never told him about. Maybe I will, someday, but right now, it just wouldn't feel right.

I first developed it when I was in college. I was addicted to poker in those days. I mean addicted. Those cards were just about all I could think about. I played almost every night, and sometimes bet a whole week's budget on a single pot. I was a good student and didn't have to waste much time studying. What's more, I was lucky. I almost always got up from the table a winner.

Anyway, one night, I was playing stud poker with four guys I knew. We used to play together fairly often, although, away from the card table, we didn't have anything to do with each other. At one point, I found myself with four queens, two of them showing and two in the hole—that means hidden from the other players. One of the guys had three eights on the table, and was strongly hinting that he had a fourth in the hole.

The betting was getting pretty heavy. Everybody was raising everybody else, and when it got to me it was a case of put up or shut up. It would have cost me about another hundred dollars to stay in the game, and I just didn't have it. It killed me, because I was holding the best hand I ever had in my life. "Hey, look," I said. "You don't want to win this by raising me out of the game, do you? How about letting me go shy a hundred. If I lose, I'll pay you back next week."

One of the guys was willing, but the others said, "No way." Then, the guy who was holding the eights said, "Tell you what. We'll let you go shy the hundred. But if you lose, you've got to put out for all of us here. If that's all right with the rest of you guys, that is."

No one objected, and neither did I, because I was that sure of winning. But first I wanted to play with the concept a little, because for some strange reason the idea kind of turned me on. "Now, wait a minute," I said. "You mean if I lose I've got to screw you all?"

"Whatever we want," one of them said. "Maybe screw; maybe blowjobs. Maybe two at a time. Whatever we want."

I looked at my cards again and said, "Okay. It's a deal." With that, I turned over my hole cards to show my four queens. The guys all groaned and threw their cards onto the table.

"Oh, it could have been so nice," one of them said. I just laughed as I scooped up the pot.

Later that night, though, I lay in bed, imagining what it would have been like to be their private poker slut, available at their whim to perform whatever sexual acts they thought might give them pleasure. It got me all hot and stimulated. Before I knew it, I was masturbating to a series of degrading images of myself as a sex slave.

I pictured removing my panties and leaving the rest of my clothes on as they lined up and lifted my skirt to take turns screwing me. One would be in me, rocking forward and back, while the rest watched and egged him on. Or maybe two of them would continue playing cards while the other two made a sandwich out of me, one entering me from in front and another in my rear.

Of course, I was younger then, and it didn't take me very long to get off. Within minutes, I was coming to the churning of my own fingertips and the swirling visions of being a slave to the poker players. After that, being a poker slut became my favorite fantasy.

In my lucid moments, I realized how close I had come to doing something really crazy that night. Poker stopped having the same attraction for me. In fact, I played very little after that, and never for really high stakes. But I still amused myself by imagining being at the complete disposal of a group of horny, poker-playing men.

It's funny, but Brady turned out to be a poker player, although never addicted the way I was. He likes to get together with some of the men he works with for games that sometimes last into the wee hours of the morning. They play about once a week, rotating from one house to another. Which means that every month or so, they come here.

That's when the poker-slave fantasy really works me up. On the night of their game, I find myself dressing provocatively, wearing low-cut tops that show my breasts when I bend over even slightly. Then, while they play, I take care of the table. I bring them beers and sandwiches, empty the ashtrays, clear the dishes. Anything to give me a chance to be at the table and expose myself casually to them. Sometimes, I wear a real short skirt so that whenever I have to pick something up off the floor, they can see my panties. They try to hide it, but I know they are looking.

Then I go into my room and fantasize. I imagine that Brady is losing heavily. Finally, with nothing else to bet, he agrees that if he loses the next hand, they can all use me any way they want. They argue about it for a while, trying to decide whether his offer is worth the pot that he's betting into. Brady makes me come out and stand before them so they can look me over while they decide. He even makes me take off some of my clothes.

I imagine standing there in my brief bra and panties while the men stare at me and lick their lips, thinking about the things they'll get to do to me if Brady loses the hand. One of them calls me over and strokes my thigh, as if testing the merchandise. Another reaches his fingers inside my bra and touches my erect nipple, while a third pats my ass. Finally, they agree to the bet, and the last card is dealt.

I stand there and watch as Brady turns over his hand. He's got a straight to the ten, and I'm confident he's going to win. He beats two pairs. And he beats a low straight. But one of the men has a flush. And another has a full house. Everyone laughs raucously. Everyone except Brady.

"All right, Cynthia," he says quietly. "A bet's a bet."

For a moment all is silent. Then the one with the full house says, "I'm the winner, so I guess I ought to get first dibs. Come over here and suck my cock."

Hesitantly, I walk toward him, with no choice but to obey. I stand in front of him for a moment, waiting for him to open his pants, but he says, "No, take off all your clothes first. We want to see everything you've got."

I feel my face reddening as their gaze centers on me. I start to reach back for the clip that holds my bra shut. I feel Brady's fingers there ahead of mine, twisting and unhooking it to allow my breasts to swing forward for all to see. One of the men reaches up and casually pinches my nipples, first the left then the right. Everyone laughs again.

"Now the panties," someone says. "And nobody help her. We want to see her do it herself." I am embarrassed by their stares as I hook my thumbs into the elastic waistband and start to draw the wispy garment slowly down over my hips. When I feel my dark pubic hair coming into view, I know that I've reached the point of no return. It's quiet in the room, all the men concentrating on the spectacle I'm making of myself. The only sound I can hear is heavy breathing.

Finally, I am totally naked, completely exposed to their lustful stares. I am at their beck and call, with no will of my own. Full-house says, "That blowjob. I want it now. Take out my cock."

While everyone watches, I drop to my knees in front of him and begin fumbling with the front of his pants. I can feel his erection straining against the material and I can see a little wet dot where it is oozing with excitement. I get his pants open, but he makes no move to stand up. I'm going to have to suck him off with his trousers on.

Without further ceremony, I take his swollen cock in my mouth. It tastes salty and warm. I hear the men who are watching groan as I swallow half its length. I think I can recognize Brady's voice among them. I feel fingers tightening in my hair and hands moving my head up and down in a quick sexual rhythm. My eyes close tightly, but I can feel the stares of the other men on me as I perform fellatio on this relative stranger. When he comes, I have no choice but to swallow every drop of it, licking and sucking to make sure he's empty.

Then I stand, ready for the next one. Now Brady steps forward and lifts me up in his arms like a child. Another man has cleared the table. Brady lays me on it, carefully spreading my legs so that my open pussy is exposed for all to see. "Here," he says. "Who's next? Try screwing her right here on the table. You're going to like it. She's a great fuck."

One of the men opens his belt and drops his pants around his ankles. "I'll do it," he says. Roughly, he sticks his fingers into my slit and shoves them in and out. I am flowing with moisture, and this makes him laugh. "She's loving this," he says.

With the fingers of one hand, he holds my pussy lips apart, showing everyone the wet pink membranes inside. With his other hand, he grips his cock and thrusts it up against me. As I feel him sinking into my vagina, I hear the men murmuring approval. "Yeah," one of them says. "Fuck her good. Warm her up for the rest of us."

The cock is buried deep inside me now, pushing in and out until I can feel the tip of it bumping against my cervix. I feel like I'm going to come, but I'm not sure if that's permitted. Then, unable to hold it back anymore, I just let it go, moaning gutturally as the orgasm washes over me. I can feel him fucking and fucking and fucking, without stopping or even slowing down. Finally, he has fucked me so long that I feel like I'm going to come again. Only this time, he comes with me. I can feel his cock swelling and throbbing as it pumps his semen deep inside my belly.

When he's done, another man takes his place. This one turns me over so that I'm facedown on the table. He presses the tip of his penis against my pussy and then shoves it in to replace the void left by his predecessor. At the same time, another man comes to the head of the table and stands there with his cock just an inch or two from my mouth. I start nibbling it and then take the whole length in, running my tongue over it in rhythm to the movements of the cock in my pussy.

I come again. And again. And the men come too. In my mouth, in my pussy, even in my anus. I can feel their hot spunk on the cheeks of my ass, on my thighs, on my breasts, in my hair, all over my body. Until finally, all are satisfied.

For a long time I just lie there on the card table, breathing deeply as I slowly recover from the multiple fucking I have received. I look up to see Brady, smiling with approval and gratitude. His own cock is hanging down his leg to show that he too availed himself of my services while I was playing the frenzied poker slave.

Usually, by this time, I have masturbated to two or even three orgasms. Sometimes I wonder whether the men playing cards in the next room can hear me. Of course, I find myself hoping that they can. They'll never imagine what I've been thinking, though, or the part that they played in my poker-slut fantasy.

I'm sure you can see why I've never told any of this to Brady. Lately, even that's become part of the fantasy. I imagine telling him all about it and having him get so excited that he actually agrees to set it up the next time the guys come to our house for a poker game. It'll never happen of course, but just thinking about it keeps me stimulated.

Prison

Although he is only thirty-four years old, Blair wears a slightly haggard look that makes him appear older than his years. Beneath it all, though, are handsome Irish features. His black hair is tousled in a way that makes women want to run their fingers through it. His blue eyes twinkle as he speaks, smiling even when his full lips do not. He is five feet eleven inches tall and of medium build. One of his muscled arms bears a crude tattoo, the word MINE in shaky capital letters.

I hate this fucking tattoo and I'll have to wear it my whole life. My cell mate put it on me with a sharpened piece of metal and some ink from a ballpoint pen. That's when I was in prison. All because of a couple of beers too many.

I never thought of alcohol as a problem. I love it and it loves me. I can hold it better than most men. All the fucking law cares about is the numbers, though. The second time I got arrested for driving under the influence, my numbers were too fucking high. Point one eight is what they said. Point one fucking eight.

So what, I says. It didn't affect my driving. Six months, says the judge. And off they led me, like a common fucking criminal. My wife just stood there weeping. "Don't worry, darlin'," I told her. "I'll be home before you know it."

Some people do murders and don't get six months. I served every last fucking day of the sentence. I used to make decent wages as a welder. Now I'm lucky to get work as a handyman. I'm an ex-con is what I am. Once you have a record, you're done for. Nobody wants you.

Prison was a bitch. I figured they'd put me in some low-security facility with other minor offenders like myself. But I ended up in a cell with a fucking first-class career criminal. An armed robber who spent more of his life behind bars than on the outside. He was a huge fucker. Everybody called him "Big Jim" or just plain "Big." A real monster of a man, inside and out.

I knew I was in trouble the second they put me in the cell with him. He looked at me with beady little eyes and half a smile on his face. I could feel him checking me up and down the way a man might check a woman, and I started to sweat. "Oh, I'm going to have fun with you," the bastard said.

I've had my share of fights in my lifetime. One thing I've learned is that once you let someone intimidate you, you're his slave for life. So, without waiting another second, I hauled off and punched Mister Big right in the mouth. He thereupon proceeded to beat the living shit out of me.

Even after it was obvious that I had lost, he kept kicking and pummeling me as I lay helpless on the concrete floor of the cell. I yelled for help, but I might as well have asked the clouds to carry me off to heaven. Big Jim just laughed and said, "You're mine, you little prick. You're going to do what-ever I want."

He was kind enough to wait about fifteen minutes for the blood to stop gushing from my nose and broken lips before he grabbed my hair and yanked me to my knees. Without ceremony, he opened the front of his pants and took out his dick, which was huge like the rest of him. It was erect and swollen. I guess kicking my ass had turned him on. "Now suck this," he ordered.

I hesitated, but only long enough for him to swing his hamlike hand and crack me a good one across the face. He placed his hand at the back of my head and pushed my lips against the tip of his cock. I had no choice but to open my mouth and let him in. "Suck it," he commanded again. "And don't think of biting me or I'll tear your fucking head off." I knew he meant it and that he could do it as easy as breaking a lead pencil. So I did as he said.

For the first time in my life, I sucked a man's cock. It filled my whole mouth and nudged at the opening of my throat, almost making me gag. I was afraid of what he would do if I started retching, so I fought the reflex and held back the throat spasms. His fingers tangled in my hair, he pumped my head back and forth until I felt his cock getting even bigger inside my mouth. "You better fucking swallow every drop," he snarled as it started to spit into my throat. What else could I do?

The fucker made me give him blowjobs every day for the next week. It didn't matter to him if other prisoners were watching through the bars, or even if there were guards walking down the rows. Everybody seemed to be afraid of him. The fucking officials ignored what was going on. I was a sex slave. Period.

For the first few days, he beat me up every time before forcing me to do what he wanted. He said he was training me, domesticating me. After a while, he stopped punching me around. He'd just snap his fingers and point to his crotch. It was my job to unbutton his fly; take out his prick, get on my knees, and suck it until he was satisfied. I gave up trying to resist. It was hopeless. I was helpless.

After about a week, the blowjobs stopped satisfying him. "Turn around and bend over," he muttered one night. "I'm going to fuck you in the ass." The idea horrified me, but I knew there was no point in putting up a fight. All that would happen was he'd beat me half to death and then have his way with me anyway. So, docilely, I obeyed his command.

I'll never forget that first time. He made me take off my pants and underwear. He fondled my cock for a minute with his rough, callused hand. Then he turned me around and started rubbing my asshole with his finger. "Here," he said. "I'll let you wet my cock so it won't hurt so much when I take your cherry." He was doing me a fucking favor, you see.

He stood there like a lord while I licked his cock all over like he directed me to. Then he turned me around again and had me put my hands on the lower bunk. I felt the head of his dick working its way between the cheeks of my ass, seeking my tight little asshole. Without any further ado, he shoved it in.

I don't think anything ever hurt so much in my whole life. I could feel every fucking millimeter of his giant prick forcing its way inside. I couldn't help crying out, but when I did, he whacked the back of my head with his open hand. "Shut up, bitch," he said. "You'll learn to love it before too long."

He gave me another whack for good measure and then started sawing in and out of me, fucking me the way a man fucks a woman. Oh, it hurt, but I bit my lip and took it. The thought of him spewing his hot disgusting sperm into my asshole positively made me sick, but I knew it was going to happen. When it did, I could feel every throbbing spasm of his cock as it reared up and spit again and again.

He kept shoving it in and out until he was completely empty. Then he let it slip out of me with a plopping sound and pushed me forward onto the bed. I just lay there in silence, my ass feeling like it was on fire. I couldn't imagine how I'd get through five and a half more months of this slavery.

I knew he'd be doing it again and I didn't want it to be as painful as that first experience had been. I wished there was some way I could get some Vaseline, but I had no idea how to go about doing that. The next morning at breakfast, I got hold of a chunk of margarine and wrapped it in a scrap of cloth that I tore off my handkerchief. Big Jim saw what I was doing and grinned malevolently. "You're a good boy," he said.

Later, back in the cell, he said, "Grease up your ass, bitch. I'm ready for some more." I did as he told me, grateful that he was allowing me the opportunity to do something to ease the pain. I worked the margarine into my asshole before bending over to let him at me. The second time was a lot easier than the first, either because of the grease, or because I had been so stretched, or both.

The third time he did it to me, a strange thing happened. Oh, it still hurt, but it felt a little bit good, too. I didn't understand it. In fact, I was too busy trying not to cry out to even give it any thought. There's no doubt that there was a pleasant sensation mixed with the pain, though. His words, "You'll learn to love it before too long," kept running through my head as he fucked my ass until he came. At one point, I almost felt like I would come, myself.

The next time, I actually did come. He was pumping away inside of me, driving his cock in and out for all he was worth, when suddenly, without any fucking warning, my cock rose up and started to shoot. I couldn't fucking believe it. My asshole still hurt, but not nearly as much as before.

After that, it seemed like the more he did it to me, the less it hurt. Awful as it is to say, I came every single time. Not only was I his slave, but I was starting to become a willing slave. It's hard for me to face this, but the orgasms I got when he fucked me in the ass got to be more intense than any orgasms I could ever remember having with my wife or any other woman. Was prison making me gay?

Once I started to come from getting fucked in the ass, the cell didn't seem quite so much like hell anymore. At least not physically. Now I was tormented by the thought of what I was becoming. He didn't leave me much time for thinking about that, though, because in between fucking me in the ass, he was starting to make me suck him off again. No matter how many times I did that, I always hated it. To my horror, there were even times I found myself asking him, begging him, to fuck me instead. Oh, he really liked that. He would laugh and laugh, the dirty bastard.

The state must have been making examples of drunk drivers, because I was in for the full six months. But a day finally came when my time was up and I was scheduled to be released. I waited until I heard the guards coming down the hall to get me out of my cell. Then, at the very last minute,

I gave Big Jim one good solid kick in the balls. I put the entire weight of my body behind that kick, and all the rage that had been building in me since that first day I became his prisoner. He fell to the floor and lay there writhing, both hands clutching his groin, as the guards led me away. As a final good-bye, I called, "Fuck you," over my shoulder.

My wife was waiting to take me home. Let me tell you, she was a sight for sore fucking eyes. Mine filled up with tears at the first glimpse of her. You might think that after what I'd been through I'd be craving sex with her, or dying for certain foods, or maybe a drink. It wasn't like that at all. When we got home, I slept for two whole days. For the first time in six months, I didn't have to worry that my monster of a cell mate would wake me up to put it to me.

I was very disturbed about the way I had reacted to being fucked by him. For more than a week, I couldn't bring myself to touch my wife. Finally, she started looking at me funny, so I had to make myself do it. The last fucking thing in the world I'd ever want would be for her to know that for six months I was the sex slave of a fucking armed robber known as Big Jim.

That first sex session with her was okay, but not as good as it should have been. Things didn't get any better, though. After a while, my wife began to get really worried about me. She asked me to talk to her about prison and what I had experienced there, but I just couldn't bring myself to do it. Finally, she insisted that I see a doctor, a psychiatrist. She said I owed it to her, if not to myself. So I agreed.

It wasn't until the third visit that I made myself tell the doc about the things Big Jim had made me do and the things he had done to me. The doctor listened for a while without saying a word. Then he said, "You had orgasms, didn't you? And now you're worried that you might be homosexual." I guess he had experience with men who had been to prison.

When he said this, I actually started to cry. He handed me a box of tissues and let me use them. When I settled down a bit, he explained that my response was purely physiological. It has been proven, he said, that massage of the prostate gland will produce intense orgasms in any man. The only way to reach the prostate is through the rectum. He told me that when law enforcement officials need a semen sample from a rape suspect who refuses to provide it, they get it by shoving a gloved finger up his ass and massaging the prostate. He said it works every fucking time.

Prison hadn't turned me homosexual, after all. It had just exposed me to an experience that I might not otherwise have had. After that, I felt different about the whole thing. Now, instead of being turned off by the thought of getting fucked in the ass, I get turned on by it. Sometimes I wish I could tell my wife all about it and get one of those dildo things that women use on themselves to have her use it on me.

I'd never want her to know about the things Big Jim made me do. I couldn't stand having her picture me bent over the bunk while that huge fucker made me come by digging his stiff prick into my asshole. How could she ever respect me if she knew about that?

SEVEN
Garment Fetish

*S*ome people have a tendency to connect sexuality with certain kinds of garments. This has been called "fetishism," but naming a tendency does little to explain it. Psychologists offer theories, most of which we find to be unsatisfactory.

Take the notorious foot fetish, for example. Freud said that our earliest sexual experiences occur while we are infants. Infants spend a great deal of time crawling around on the floor among shod grown-up feet. By coincidence, dragging the genitals along a carpeted or smooth wooden surface may produce a juvenile orgasm at the precise moment that a child happens to be looking at a woman's high-heeled shoe. If this occurs, some writers claim, the child probably will grow up with an erotic preoccupation with women's feet and footwear.

Frankly, we don't buy this theory. For one thing, it fails to explain why no one ever seems to be turned on by men's footwear. The sight of a wingtip or balmoral leaves most people cold. For another, it does not even begin to provide reasons for other popular clothing fetishes.

One of these involves a fascination with leather. Most suppliers of erotic paraphernalia offer selections of leather garments that are obviously designed to be sexually stimulating. Briana, a woman whose story is told in this chapter, remembers the leather fetish of her recent rebellious youth and still finds the thought of it arousing.

Rock speaks of an erotic attachment to women's panties. The proliferation of lingerie calendars and similar pop art suggests that this preoccupation is not unusual. However, Rock admits that when he sees a woman wearing them, he is less interested in her than in the undergarment she has on.

We will not attempt to offer any explanation for the attractions our informants describe. We are content to recognize that such feelings exist, without understanding why, and to pass on to our readers our recognition of that reality. To some extent, however, we do comprehend why the desires these people describe remain unspoken.

Leather

$\mathcal{A}$t twenty-one, Briana is the picture of modern conservative womanhood. She is tall and slim, with an air of self-
assuredness that comes from having all material needs
satisfied. Her chestnut hair is shoulder-length, worn in a style
that could come right out of the pages of *Vogue* or *Made-
moiselle*. Her light brown eyes look steadily into those of
whomever she is facing, reinforcing the sense of confidence
that she exudes. Her white teeth are perfectly straight. She
is not employed, but spends several hours a day tending to
the family fortune.

I guess you would say that I was born with the proverbial
silver spoon in my mouth. My family's money is old. As an
only child, I always had everything I wanted. Except my parents' attention. From my earliest memories, they traveled all
over the world, leaving me to the care of a nurse or a nanny
and a house full of servants.

As I grew older, I found myself resenting this more and
more. When they would return temporarily from their trav-
els, I was extremely belligerent and defiant. By my early
teens, I was rebelling against them in every way I could think
of. I did whatever I knew would hurt them and offend their
way of life.

They tried sending me off to boarding schools, but nothing
they could do would keep me there. In spite of the huge
amounts of money they paid, I would be expelled for lack of

discipline. If that didn't happen, I would run away and disappear for a while. Eventually, my parents had no choice but to hire private tutors to come to our house and instruct me.

By the time I was sixteen, I was far too much for anyone to handle. Maybe that's why my parents seemed to be traveling even more than before. Now they would only come home on special holidays. Between times, the servants they employed had sole responsibility for me.

The less time they spent with me, the more resentful of them I became. I developed a burning desire to get back at them for all the crimes and misdemeanors I thought they had committed against me. I just couldn't wait to get out from under their control—legal if not actual. When I turned eighteen, I got my chance.

That's when I started receiving income from a trust that was left to me by my mother's parents. I had plenty of money of my own now and felt I needed no one. I left the palatial family home behind, and with it the conservative lifestyle in which I had grown up. Filled with anger and seeking ways of getting back at my parents, I cultivated a strange bunch of new friends.

We were a loosely organized band of motorcyclists, traveling together from place to place, from state to state. All the members were rebels, like me. They came from many different backgrounds. Some were from the middle class. Others had grown up on the streets. What all of us had in common was a devotion to something we called "freedom" and a sense of nonconformity. We got up when we liked. We ate when we were hungry. We moved on when we got tired of a place. We had sex whenever we felt like it and with whomever we happened to be at the moment.

We identified ourselves with leather jackets that had the words "Live for the Road" emblazoned on the backs. Beneath the jackets, we wore leather vests. We also wore leather pants, leather hats, leather gloves, and leather boots. The women all wore leather bras, either under their clothing or right out in front where they could be seen. Under my pants, I wore a leather G-string that barely covered my privates, except when I took it off to give one, or two, or more of the men, and some of the women, access to my willing vagina.

Sometimes we'd have parties at which we all dressed in leather fetish garments. It was like a continual contest to see who could come up with the most outrageously erotic leather outfit. My personal favorite was a corset that was tightly laced in the front. It was constructed in a way that showed my nipples, pushing my breasts up and together, to make them look huge and to create a sharp cleavage between them. It was open at the bottom, showing much of my pubic hair framing the leather G-string. Some of the women wore harnesses that encircled and exposed their breasts, causing them to stand out like cannons ready for battle. The leather was always black and usually decorated with big silver studs.

A lot of the men donned leather jockstraps. Others sported penis sheaths, like studded shrouds around their organs, forcing all the blood to the swollen purple heads so they would stay erect for hours. One of the men would wear nothing but a series of five or six leather rings around his penis, about an inch apart, so tight that the flesh would swell up and turn red between them. On a few occasions, we took group photos, all dressed in our leathers. I'd send them to my parents just for the shock value.

We'd drink ourselves into a state of oblivion at those parties. Then the orgies would begin. Sometimes I'd have sex with three or four different men, one right after the other, or even all at the same time. All around me, those who weren't similarly occupied would be cheering us on. I'd see women with women, men with men, and groups made up of every imaginable combination. Sometimes, I'd be so intoxicated that I wouldn't even know if the people who were playing with my body were male or female. I might find myself holding a vagina in one of my hands and a penis in the other, with another in my mouth, and yet another inside me.

The fetish garments were very much part of the erotic

mystique. Something about the feel of the leather, the smell of it, even the taste of it, would add spice to the sexual stimulation. It seemed quite natural for us to strut around in our erotic finery, showing ourselves off, turning ourselves and each other on, and then indulging our most twisted and perverted desires. I don't think it would have worked without the leather.

I remember one weekend we all rode to an isolated glade in the forest, somewhere in the Rocky Mountains. It was summer, and the air was redolent with the smell of sex. We all got drunk, put on our leather garments, and started to play. Someone got the idea of voting on who was wearing the sexiest outfit. The winner would get to have sex with everyone there.

We all wanted the prize, so we went to great lengths to make whatever we had on look even more alluring by placing flowers in strategic places or leaving buttons undone. I loosened the laces of my leather corset so that most of my body was uncovered and I inserted a big white wild flower in my vulva. I stuck a bundle of little purple blossoms in my cleavage and a series of bright red blooms between the open laces. I wove a bunch of yellow daisies into a crown that I wore on my head.

When my turn came to stand on the tree stump that we were using for a stage, the crowd went wild. The men cat-called; the women were hooted and applauded. I was proclaimed the winner.

The group formed a circle around me and started moving in closer and closer to give me my prize. My head was spinning from a combination of alcohol and erotic excitement. There were at least thirty people there. Every one of them was going to have a turn with me.

We all kept our leather garments on as one by one they stepped up to where I was waiting and did things to me. One of the men wearing a penis sheath masturbated by rubbing the head of his organ until he covered my exposed breasts with his semen. Another fell to his knees and began performing cunnilingus on my waiting vulva. When he was done, another bent me over and assaulted my anus with his swollen member.

The women participated, too, licking and sucking my genitals, playing with my breasts, inserting fingers and tongues in every possible opening of my body. I had one orgasm after another, until I was totally spent. But there was no stopping the parade of revelers. The sex continued until every one of them had satisfied him- or herself in, or on, or with my body. I don't know how long it lasted. When we started, the sun was high in the sky. When the orgy wound down, the moon was shining its pale light on us.

Somehow, that forest bacchanal was a turning point. Maybe it was because after that there was nothing left for me to do. I had already tried everything. More likely, it was because of a telegram that finally reached me about three weeks after it was sent. Both my parents had been killed in the crash of a private plane somewhere in Africa.

I had to go back home, at least for a while, to set the family's financial affairs in order. I told my friends and myself that I would return when I finished taking care of business. Deep down, though, I must have known I wouldn't. Before the group accompanied me to the airport, I signed my motorcycle over to one of the other women who always rode on the back of a guy's bike because she didn't have wheels of her own.

I didn't really know how wealthy my family was until I met with the lawyers and started going over the books. It was amazing. Suddenly, I felt a sense of responsibility. Someone had to manage all these assets. There was no one to do it but me. It wasn't long before I became educated about the world of finance and began taking charge.

I couldn't have done it without help, of course. That came from Kent. He was a professional money manager who had made quite a reputation on Wall Street, even though he was less than thirty years old. My parents had first consulted him about a year before their death. Now I became his only client.

As Kent and I worked closely together, I learned quite a lot about him. While I had been to the manner born, Kent was completely self-made and proud of it. He came from a lower-middle-class family. He had attended Harvard on a full academic scholarship. Then he worked his way up from junior stockbroker to an advisor of millionaires.

He knew about my upbringing and even about my years of teenage rebellion. But he had no idea of my escapades with the motorcycle group. There wasn't any way I could tell him.

I developed a respect for him that soon ripened into love. We are engaged and expect to be married within a few months. We have great sex. I've even gone so far as to get a tiny leather G-string that I wear for him on special occasions. No studs. Probably it excites me more than it does him.

I don't exactly miss the old crowd or the crazy irresponsible things we did. I do miss the leather fetish garments, though. They made me feel like there was nothing in the world but sex; nothing to do but play erotic games from morning till night.

I'm certain Kent would never understand any of that. He'd be a little afraid of that much or that kind of freedom. It would turn him off, instead of turning him on.

Occasionally, I come across a fetish-wear catalog and leaf through it, remembering the feeling I used to get in my leather corset, looking at men in their cock rings and penis sheaths. I've even thought of buying some leather outfits and wearing them secretly, when I'm home alone, to get myself turned on for sex with Kent later on. But I've given up that life and I just have to learn to face it. I'm a Republican now. People of my class don't do such things.

Panties

$\mathcal{T}$he man described in this story insisted that we identify him by his nickname, Rock. He says that everyone calls him that. Rock is forty-five years old and about five feet eleven inches tall. He is on the corpulent side, weighing in at around two hundred ten pounds, very little of which is muscle. He wears his salt-and-pepper hair cropped close to his head. His eyes are steely gray. Rock is employed as part of the maintenance crew in a complex of college dormitories.

It ain't the best-paying job in the world, but it's steady. I got a good retirement plan and great medical and dental insurance. The best part is the panties benefits. See, panties have always done it for me, as long as I can remember.

I couldn't have been more than four or five the first time I really noticed a woman in panties. It was my aunt, my mother's sister. She was staying with us. Because I was a little kid, she didn't pay much attention when I walked in and out of her room while she was dressing.

One day I caught her in nothing but bra and panties. The second I saw her, I felt the strangest sensation go through my body. I wasn't all that interested in the bra, but I just couldn't take my eyes off the panties and the way they hugged her crotch. It was obvious she wasn't shaped like I was, or my daddy. I was aware that ladies had boobies and men didn't. But I never realized there was such a difference down below. Somehow, I was less interested in what was inside the panties as I was in the panties themselves.

I ran to my aunt and threw my arms around her for a hug, like I did lots of times, only this time with an ulterior motive. When I hugged her, I pressed my face against her panties. I'm sure it seemed natural to her, because that's how tall I was. How could she know that I was inhaling deeply to treat my nostrils to that female fragrance that has haunted me all the rest of my life?

After that, it seemed that my mind was constantly filled with images of panties and memories of that sweet, spicy scent. On Sundays, I would leaf through the newspaper, page by page. My parents thought I was looking at the comic strips, but I was really searching for lingerie ads featuring panties. Whether they were shown alone or on drawings of models, they simply fascinated me.

When I got into my early teens, the ads in newspapers weren't enough for me. Like the rest of my friends, I looked at plenty of *Playboy* magazines. The other guys all talked about the big boobs and hairy pussies, but I was dissatisfied, because there weren't enough pictures of women in panties. I actually preferred Frederick's of Hollywood catalogs.

By the time I was fifteen or so, I started my collection of panties. I would go out at night and prowl the neighborhood, looking for women's underwear hanging on clotheslines. I'd climb over fences or jump over hedges to get into the yards and steal pairs of them. Later, I'd take them home and fondle them while beating off. Sometimes I'd rub my cock with the panties themselves, shooting my adolescent load right into them.

Around Mother's Day or Christmas, I'd browse through the lingerie departments of big stores, pretending to be shopping for a gift for my mother. In reality, I'd be looking at the panties. I handled them, too, whenever I got a chance. I even bought a few pairs and added them to my collection.

I still wasn't satisfied. That glorious scent I had first experienced with my face pressed against my auntie's crotch continued to haunt me. My aunt didn't spend much time with us anymore, or I would have tried to find a way of getting into her laundry basket. I wished I had an older sister, just for that reason. On a couple of occasions, I thought of going through my mother's dirty clothes, looking for her worn panties. But the guilt was more than I could handle.

When I first started dating, I was different from other guys my age. All they could dream of was getting their hands on a girl's tits and maybe someday getting into their panties. I was just interested in the panties themselves. If I could see them, I had triumphed. If I could touch them, I was in heaven. Oh, God, if only I could figure out a way to smell them.

I got my own apartment when I was nineteen. Things were freer then. AIDS hadn't been invented yet. I brought lots of girls home for sex, even though screwing them really wasn't my ultimate goal. It was something I had to do just to get a shot at the panties.

I would feel their pussies for a long time before undressing them, to be sure the panties got good and wet. Then, when the girl wasn't looking, I'd kick them under the bed. We'd look all over for them, unsuccessfully, and finally she'd have to go home without them. As soon as she left, I'd put them into a zipper-lock bag to preserve the fragrance.

Later, when I was alone, I'd take them out of the bag and sniff the wet crotch while jerking my cock. The lingering scent of pussy musk never failed to bring me up and get me off. Every girl's panties smelled different. I found that if I put them back in the plastic bag right after using them, they would stay fragrant for weeks. Finally, when the smell was almost gone, I'd take the crotch in my mouth and suck out whatever flavor lingered in the material.

I had to support myself through all this, so I worked at various jobs. Nothing very exciting, just enough to keep a roof over my head and food in my mouth. I never was the studious kind, so high school was the end of my education. Fortunately, my wants were very small.

Then, a friend of my father's recommended me for a job that was right up my alley. It's the job I've had for the past twenty-plus years. I'm in the maintenance department for all the dormitories at the college. Half of them are for boys, or young men, I guess. The other half are for young women.

In the men's dorm, I just fix the pipes, or patch up holes in the walls, or take care of general wear and tear. In the women's, I get to go on panty hunts. There were a few times when I was fixing the shower or something that I actually got to see a couple of girls in panties. But I'm much more interested in the panties than in the girls.

When repairs have to be made, I have free access to the rooms, as long as there's nobody in them. That gives me a wealth of underpants to choose from. You'd be surprised at what slobs these young ladies can be now that they're away from home and living on their own. Lots of times, I find dirty clothes piled all over the floor, or on the beds, including worn underwear.

I love to go through the piles, handling each pair of panties that I find. I examine the crotch for discoloration, thinking of all the things that make a young woman's juices flow. I sniff the sweet fragrance of budding young pussy on one pair after another. Sometimes, when two girls share a room, I can tell which panties belong to one and which belong to another by the difference in scent.

If the women are a little neater, I look for whatever it is they keep their laundry in. I'm always sure to find worn panties in there. Sometimes, those are even better, because being in a basket or a bag sort of concentrates the fragrance, so that by the time I get my nose into them, they smell so strong and sweet that a couple of sniffs is enough to get my cock all hard and throbbing.

Then what I like to do is get a clean pair out of their bureau and jerk off into it. I wrap it around my cock and rub myself up and down until I come all over the crotch. Cotton is best because it absorbs the liquid right away. When they're dry, I refold them neatly and place them back where I found them. Later, I imagine the girl wearing those panties with my cum right up against her wide-open, naked pussy. The thought of it drives me nuts.

If I come across a particularly fragrant pair of worn ones, I take it with me to play with later on. I carry zipper-lock bags with me just for that purpose. I have more than three hundred pairs of worn panties in my collection. I keep them locked away in my tool chest in the garage so my wife won't find them.

Oh, yeah, maybe I didn't mention I'm married. My wife likes to wear pretty panties and she knows I like seeing her in them. But she would never understand that it's the panties themselves that turn me on. That's just not the kind of thing a man can explain to his wife. She'd probably think I'm some kind of freak.

Once, I took a pair of her worn panties out of the laundry basket and put them in a plastic bag to save the smell. Then I took them to a lingerie shop, removing them from the plastic just before going inside. There was a young woman working behind the counter. When she said, "Can I help you?" I showed her the panties.

I told her that they were my wife's and said that I wanted to get her some more just like them. I asked if she had the same kind. She took them from me and held them up to the light to get a good look at them. Then she brought them close to her face so she could read the words on the little label sewn into the waistband.

I knew she could see the discoloration in the crotch and I'm sure she could smell the spicy musk of my wife's pussy. Watching her handle those panties and knowing that her nostrils were filling with their fragrance gave me an instant hard-on. Good thing I was standing by the counter where she couldn't see it.

I asked her if she could tell me what kind of material they were made of and watched as she rubbed the cloth between her thumb and forefinger. It just happened to be the crotch that she was holding. That made me even hotter. She lifted them up for another look at the label before telling me they were a rayon blend.

She said she didn't have another pair just like it but offered to show me some similar ones. I let her take six or seven different kinds off the shelf before saying, No, I wanted to find some just like the ones I had brought in. The fact was I needed to get away from there before I creamed my jeans from seeing her handling and smelling my wife's underpants along with all those fresh ones. I went straight from the store to the men's room, where I relieved myself by jerking off into my wife's worn panties.

I realize my little fetish may be unusual, but it's harmless enough. I sure wish my wife understood it. Just imagine the games we could play together if she did. For example, I'd ask her to wear the same pair for a week, so that it would get really pungent. Then I'd have her watch me jerk off while sniffing them. Or maybe, on her own, she'd put a pair of worn panties in my lunchbox one morning, so I'd be surprised by it in the middle of the day. Jeez, imagine if I could ask her to get me some other woman's panties to play with.

I know good and goddamn well that's a pipe dream. It ain't never going to happen. I'll just have to play the panty games by myself. I guess that ain't so bad.

EIGHT
Cross-Dressing

Cross-dressing has drawn quite a bit of media attention, lately. There have even been lawsuits by male public employees demanding the right to dress in female clothing. The public outcry is sometimes astonishing. Cross-dressers occasionally become the victims of hate crimes, although why anyone should become so violently emotional about the clothing someone else chooses to wear is beyond our understanding.

Despite what most people think, the desire to dress in garments of the opposite gender is not always related to homosexuality. Many men who lead perfectly ordinary sex lives have admitted to us that they sometimes wear women's panties under their business suits. They say they like the way the silky material feels against their masculine organs.

The male cross-dresser who tells his story in this chapter is heterosexual and married. He first experimented with women's clothing because a girlfriend promised that she would give him a special sexual treat if he would indulge her in this fashion. Even though he pretended to flirt with other men, he was never sexually attracted to them and did nothing to compromise his heterosexuality.

Society does not regard cross dressing by women as a problem. Female fashions often include garments, like trousers, jackets, shirts, and ties, that are modeled after those traditionally worn by men. Colleen, whose story is also told in this chapter, carries her cross dressing one step further, however. Taking advantage of her boyish figure, she actually masquerades as a young male, wearing a man's bathing suit on her trips to the beach and going shirtless on public streets. She, too, is heterosexual, never even hinting at a sexual interest in members of her own gender.

After the initial nervousness wore off, neither was personally uncomfortable about cross dressing. Neither feared that their pleasure at wearing garments designed for members of the opposite gender reflected on their own sexuality. However, both were unwilling to divulge to the person with whom they share their lives their history of having experienced this pleasure. If they had not told us, their desire would remain forever unspoken.

The Dress-up Game

_L_ynn, who is in his mid-thirties, owns a family-style lunch and dinner restaurant. He says he's been in the restaurant business since he was a teenager, working for his parents until they retired. He took over the restaurant just a few years ago. He is tall and thin, with fine blond hair that is cut close on the sides and longer in the back. His gray eyes seem to be appraising everything they see. His fair skin is clear and almost translucent.

My wife calls me "pretty boy" sometimes, because of my complexion. She has no idea how pretty I can be. We were both over thirty when we met. We only knew each other a few months before we got married. I'm sure neither one of us have told the other one everything.

We're very compatible in every way, including sex. She's kind of conventional, though. Our sex is kind of conventional, too. I guess I prefer it that way. Between you and me, the most exciting sex I can remember was with this kinky girlfriend I once had named Maris. I ended up leaving her, though.

Before I met my wife, I had my share of girlfriends. Maris was one of them. After we lived together for about five months, she turned out to be a little too weird for me. So we broke up. Man, some of the things she wanted to do, you just wouldn't believe. I mean S&M, bondage, all kinds of stuff like that. She was really off the wall. There was one little game she liked to play that turned me on, though. We called it "the dress-up game." We did it a lot.

The first time, it came as a complete surprise to me. It was a Monday and the restaurant was closed. I had nothing to do but hang around the apartment thinking about screwing Maris the second she got home. When she finally came in the door, I was really hungry for her. I rushed to her and took her in my arms. She let me kiss her, but then she slipped away from me.

"Not just yet," she said. "I want you good and horny for what I have in mind."

I was already familiar with some of her wild ideas, so I asked cautiously, "What's that?"

"Go take a shower," she said. "I'll tell you all about it when you come out. I promise you're going to like it." As she spoke, she framed her crotch with both hands. The sight, combined with what it suggested and the promise she had made, turned me on even more than I already was. So I went straight into the bathroom and got into the shower.

When I came out, she was waiting with an electric shaver in her hand. "I'm going to shave your legs and arms," was all she said.

With some hesitation, I started to back off. "What's this all about?" I asked.

"Just do it for me," she crooned. "It won't hurt. I assure you it's going to be worth it."

I stood submissively while she applied the shaver to my legs. She shaved me all the way up to the crotch, but left my pubic hair alone. I'm not all that hairy anyway, and what hair there is pretty fine and fair. When she was done, my legs were as smooth as a girl's. She did the same to my arms, my armpits, and my chest. Now what? I wondered.

As if anticipating my question, she said, "I picked out some things for you to wear tonight." She led me into the bedroom, where panties, a bra, a skirt, and a blouse were laid out on the bed. "I want you to be my girlfriend Lynnie."

When I looked at the women's clothes, I felt really reluctant about participating in her weird little game. But she smiled at me so sweetly, and the look in her eyes promised such hot, hot sex, that I decided to give in. "Come on," she said softly. "Slip into these panties."

With a shrug, I took them from her outstretched hand and looked at them. They were lacy black. I had seen her wearing them many times, which usually got me real aroused. I thought, What the hell, maybe it will be exciting to have them on me. I was about the same size as she was, so I just stepped into them and began sliding them up my legs.

I looked into the mirror and found myself becoming aroused at my own reflection. I could see my cock beginning to stand up and wondered how I would get the panties over it. Somehow, I managed to tug them up until the elastic band was around my hips, and my cock and balls were completely covered. Strange, but the feel of that soft material against my skin was much more exciting than I imagined it could be.

Next she held out the bra. I slipped my arms into it and turned so she could hook the back. When I looked in the mirror this time, I had to suppress a giggle. Maris had good-sized tits. The cups, which were right for her, looked all deflated on me. She was prepared for that, too. Taking some foam-rubber shoulder pads from her drawer, she carefully stuffed them into the bra. Before I knew it, I had the body of a girl.

It was weird looking into the mirror at this girl in her underwear and getting turned on by the sight, all the time realizing that she was me. I don't know how to explain it, but it was like I belonged to both sexes at the same time. I almost wanted to feel myself up.

After she got me into the skirt and blouse, she said she was going to put some makeup on me. I nearly drew the line at that point, but I had already gone so far that it didn't seem to matter anymore. Besides, to be perfectly honest, the idea of being transformed into a woman was appealing to me in a way I can never expect anyone else to understand. And, believe me, I'm straight.

I sat in a chair while she applied foundation to the skin of my face, eye shadow to my upper lids, mascara to my lashes, pencil to my eyebrows, and bright red lipstick to my mouth. Then, like a crown, she placed a long blond wig on my head. I couldn't see the mirror while she was working on me, but when she was finished, she said, "Now, Lynnie, stand up and take a look."

I did as she instructed and was shocked by the change in my appearance. Like I said, I'm completely straight. I may not be all buffed out like a muscle man, but nobody would ever question my masculinity. Yet, there in the mirror was an attractive woman. How strange to realize that the woman was me. I told you Maris was kinky.

"Now," she said, "we can go to the meat market bar and grill, and you can get to see how the other half lives. You'll be one of my girlfriends. We'll have some fun flirting with the guys."

This stopped me in my tracks. It was one thing to cross-dress in private, to satisfy whatever weird desire had prompted her to ask me to do it. Going out that way was another matter. "Hold on a minute," I said, gathering my strength. "I'm not going anywhere. And you can be damn sure I'm not going with any guys. What the hell do you think I am?"

"I'm not asking you to take a man home," she said. "We'll just have some fun at the bar. Then, when you and I come home, I'll give you the hottest fucking you ever had."

I was already turned on more than I was willing to admit to myself. Added to that, her promise of what would happen when we got home overpowered any objections I had left. I agreed. She tried to get some high-heeled pumps on me, but they were way too small. I probably wouldn't have been able to walk in them anyway. At last, she settled for a pair of her sandals, which she rebuckled to fit my feet.

When we went out to the car, Maris opened he door on the passenger side and ushered me in. Then she got behind the wheel. As she drove toward the bar, I noticed some guys in another car looking hungrily at us. It was a very strange feeling to be on the other side of that kind of look. I've got to admit, it was kind of exciting. I kept glancing at my face in the mirror and still couldn't believe the change. I realized that if I saw a girl who looked that way, I'd probably be giving her the once-over myself.

I had never been to this particular bar before, so I had no fear of being recognized. It looked like Maris knew her way around. The bartender greeted her as if they were already acquainted and asked, "Who's your friend?"

"Lynnie," she said. "Meet Frank. Best bartender in town." I nodded, afraid that my voice would give me away if I spoke. "Frank," Maris said. "We'll have a couple of gin and tonics."

Sensing how nervous I was about my voice, Maris spoke softly to me as Frank was getting the drinks. "Don't be afraid to talk," she said. "Men dig women with husky voices. Anyway, yours can easily pass for a girl's." Under other circumstances, I might have been offended by such a remark, but at that particular point in time, it kind of thrilled me.

Two cocky young studs stepped up behind us. One said, "Can we get you ladies a drink?" Maris giggled.

"Frank is getting the drinks," she said, her voice showing a trace of sarcasm. "But you can pay for them." When the bartender brought our glasses, Maris just sort of bobbed her head in the direction of the guys.

Frank spoke directly to them. "That's twelve bucks for theirs," he said. "What about yourselves?"

The guys ordered beers and paid the tab. One sat down on the empty seat next to Maris. The other sat next to me. He introduced himself as Bob and said his friend's name was Chuck. Just because he bought me a drink, he seemed to think he had the liberty to put his arm around my shoulders. It pissed me off, but I remained passive. Out of the corner of my eye, I could see Chuck treating Maris the same way. Not only was she letting him, she seemed to like it.

Bob took some encouragement from my failure to stop him and went a little further, letting his hand dangle down in front of my shoulder, just an inch or so away from the swell of my stuffed bra. Now, this was an interesting development. He was going to cop a feel. In a way, I could relate to him, because I'd been in his situation a few times myself. I could also relate to what some of the women I had been with must have felt.

He tried to wear a casual, indifferent expression on his face as his hand dangled a little lower, pretending he didn't realize what was happening. When the tips of his fingers brushed against my artificial breast, I caught my breath and shifted my body, afraid that he would realize it was fake. He was so busy tuning in to my breath sound and body movement that he was oblivious to the stuffed bra. He thought I was egging him on. I couldn't help wondering how often I'd been fooled by falsies or padded bras.

Now he boldly cupped my left breast with his whole hand, whispering, "Mmm, what nice tits you have." I had no idea of how to handle this. I tried catching Maris's eye in the bar mirror, but she was busily engaged in conversation with Chuck. I noticed that Chuck's hand was trailing along Maris's thigh on the outside of her skirt. She was making no attempt to stop him, so I figured it was part of the game.

"You're only meeting one of them," I whispered to Bob, hoping that the whisper would hide the masculine sound of my voice. He never even noticed. Draining my glass, I added, "I have another. Why don't you say hello to that one, too?" I guess I said it because I had always dreamed about a woman saying something like that to me.

Bob's face lit up like a child's on Christmas morning. Shaking, he reached out with his other hand to cup my right breast. Before I had a chance to respond in any way, I heard Chuck ask whether we'd like another drink. At the sound of his friend's voice, almost guiltily, Bob dropped both hands to his sides and said, "Yeah, another drink sounds like a good idea."

While we waited for our drinks to come, I couldn't stop staring at the sight of my pretty face and feminine torso in the mirror before us. I liked the feel of women's clothing on me. It was luxurious and exciting. It was Maris's idea, but I realized I never would have gone through with this charade if it didn't actually appeal to me.

I was getting very turned on. I especially liked the way the softness of the panties I was wearing caressed my balls and cock. Seeing what looked like tits under the blouse I was wearing added to my arousal. I felt like reaching up and cupping them in my own hands. On impulse, I did.

I heard Bob gasp as he saw me do it. I deliberately provoked him by moving my hands slowly over my artificial curves, rolling the tips of my fingers around the spot where I imagined my nipples would have been if there really were breasts under my clothes. When Frank brought the next round, I dropped my hands, but not before he saw what I was doing. I could tell by the expression on his face that it got to him, too. Oh, men are so easy. I heard Maris chuckle. Apparently she approved of my actions.

We sat at the bar for about an hour, letting the guys buy us drinks. We also let them cop some feels. At one point, Bob had his hand on my leg and started slipping it up under my skirt. I played with the idea of letting him go all the way and watching the surprise on his face when he came to my nuts. I stopped him, though, when he was halfway up my thigh.

I don't quite know what made me do it, but I even reached out and touched his crotch. I can't describe or explain the weird kick I got out of feeling his cock jump at my touch. It gave me some kind of sense of power. I wouldn't exactly call it a sexual kick, but it was something. I guess it shows I was getting in to the game.

After things had heated up to the point where the guys wanted to leave and take us with them, Maris said, "Oh, I'm afraid Lynnie and I have to go now. We have an appointment." She smiled sweetly, but spitefully, as she said it.

Bob and Chuck were crestfallen. "You're kidding," Chuck said. "I was hoping we could . . . Well, you know."

"Maybe we can 'well . . . you know' some other time," I said, really into playing a catty, feminine role now. "Why don't you give us your phone numbers and maybe we'll call you."

Chuck whipped out a business card. Bob wrote his name and number on the back of it. He handed it to Maris, saying that he'd exchange it for ours, but she said, "Don't call us; we'll call you." Taking my cue, I got off the bar stool and followed her to the car. There, again, she helped me into the passenger seat and took the steering wheel.

"You were a very good girl," she said breathlessly, tossing Chuck's business card out the window. "I'm having a real good time with my friend Lynnie. Why don't we go get a bite to eat? Then we'll go home, and I'll give you your reward."

I was so horny that I would have liked to rush right home to our bed. Yet, I have to admit that there was a great deal of excitement in being dressed this way in public. I wasn't opposed to having it continue a little longer.

Maris drove to a diner, where we sat across the table from each other and had hamburgers. I tried to eat daintily, while Maris stared at me. "You make a very attractive woman," she said. "I can't wait to have you go down on my pussy dressed like that."

That was enough to take me over the limit. "I don't want any more of this burger," I said. "Please, can't we go home now?" Without another word, Maris paid the check and led me out to the car.

When we got home, she had me keep all the women's clothes on while she stripped completely naked and lay back on the bed. "Now, Lynnie," she said softly. "Eat me the way only another woman can."

I threw myself between her thighs and pressed my lip-sticked mouth against her pussy, trying to lick her more delicately than I usually did, trying to lick her the way I imagined a woman would. She came almost instantly, but I kept it up, licking and kissing and sucking her until she got excited all over again.

Then I stood and, while she watched me, removed the skirt and blouse. I left the bra and panties on. I returned to my place between her legs and started licking again. Suddenly, she pressed her thighs tight against both sides of my head and held me there as she poured forth her juices for the second time.

This time, when she was done, I removed my bra. I was going to take off the panties too, but she said, "Don't," and patted the bed beside her. I lay on my back as she directed. She pulled the panties partially down and to one side, letting my aching cock spring out. While I could still feel the fabric caressing my balls, she took my cock in her mouth and sucked me off. It was the most explosive orgasm I ever had in my life. A few minutes later, I was hard again and we fucked for a long, long time.

After that night, we played the dress-up game lots of times. If it had been her only kink, I think I might have stayed with her and lived happily ever after. But, like I said, there were too many other things. After a while I just couldn't hack it. So I moved out.

I had a few more girlfriends after that, before meeting my wife. I love the sex my wife and I have, but it is never as hot as what I had with Maris after a night out as her girlfriend Lynnie. I wish I could discuss it with my wife and maybe get her to try something like it with me. But that's absolutely out of the question. So I guess it will always have to remain a secret memory.

Flat Chest

*C*olleen, twenty-seven, is of medium height. She has long dark hair and almond-shaped, blue-gray eyes. She works at home, using her computer to design umbrellas. She is slim, with narrow hips, but is voluptuous from the waist up, with a large, softly rounded bosom that strains against her clinging, white, cashmere sweater.

I see you looking at my tits. I can't blame you. They're good ones, all right. They ought to be. Cost my husband, Darrel, a small fortune. He's the one that wanted them. As far as he's concerned, they were worth the money. Frankly, I wish I didn't have any boobs at all.

That's how it used to be. I was one of those women nature neglected when she was handing out breasts. I mean, I was really flat chested. I had nothing at all. Nothing but little pink nipples. They didn't even make training bras for the likes of me.

When I was a teenager, it bothered me. All the other girls were sprouting boobs, and I still looked like a kid. My mother tried to comfort me by calling me fashionably slim and telling me I was built like a model. That didn't make me feel any better. I kept hoping I would grow. Maybe I was just a late bloomer.

By my senior year of high school, I got used to the idea of being titless. I learned to be really satisfied with my body. I was able to participate in sports that big-breasted girls looked ridiculous playing. They'd be bouncing awkwardly all over the place, to the snickers of the boys on the sidelines, while I'd move gracefully. I never had to fidget with bra straps getting loose and slipping off my shoulders. I never had those ugly red marks that the other girls got from straps that strained against the heavy load of their boobs filling the cups.

Also, I know that my nipples were more sensitive than other girls'. We'd talk sometimes. You know how adolescent girls do. The others used to drive themselves crazy masturbating, trying to get the orgasms they read about in the magazines. All I had to do was stroke my nipples lightly. That would bring me to climax sometimes, even without touching my genitals at all.

Once, just after I finished high school, I was home alone and getting dressed to go out. I had come out of the shower and put on a pair of jeans. I wanted to wear a shirt that was hanging on the clothesline in the backyard. There was no one around and the yard was surrounded by a tall hedge. So I just ran out topless to get the shirt.

What a wonderful sensation. The cool breeze seemed to be caressing my bare nipples, exciting me and making them hard. Knowing that I was outside where, theoretically at least, I could be seen, added to the excitement. It felt so free. I found myself envying guys, who could walk around shirtless whenever the weather was right.

That was when I got the idea of passing myself off as a guy. At first it was just a little germ of a thought. The more I considered it, the more it grew and the better it seemed, until I decided to give it a try. The first step was getting my hair cut. Boys were wearing their hair long, too, but I knew that if mine were real short and combed in a masculine fashion, it would be easier for me to pull this off.

I thought of getting it cut at a regular barber shop, but decided that would be going too far. So I just went to the salon where I usually had my hair done and said I had decided to wear it real short for the summer. The beautician didn't think anything of it and kept cutting and cutting until I told her to stop.

When I went home, I stood in front of the mirror playing with it until I figured out a way to comb it in a very boyish manner. I used a little mousse on the sides to slick it back behind my ears. When I was done, I could even have fooled myself. My mother was startled, but shrugged it off, muttering something about the styles kids were in to.

The next day, I went to a department store and bought a man's bathing suit. A Speedo, real brief. I had to guess at the size, because I couldn't very well try it on. At home, I took off all my clothes and modeled the suit in front of the bedroom mirror. Some of my pubic hair protruded from the thigh bands, so I gave myself a bikini trim with my razor and tried it on again. The suit was meant to be tight and it clung to my body, revealing the outline of my crotch, even working its way up into my crack. It was too obvious that I was a girl.

I tried to think of a way of fixing that. I remembered hearing jokes about boys who stuffed socks in their swim trunks to make bulges that would make them look really hung. If it worked for them, it ought to work for me. I took a pair of sweat socks from my drawer and shoved them into the front of the suit. It was perfect. Looked just like a man's basket.

I studied myself in profile and then full front. I appeared to be a boy, all right. A skinny one, I suppose, with effeminate thighs and no hair on his chest. But there are plenty of boys who look like that. I was confident that I could pass for one of them.

We lived a few blocks from the beach, but I didn't want to try the masquerade in my own neighborhood. Somebody I knew might see me. That would really be embarrassing. So I decided to take the bus to another beach, several miles away.

I put a pair of jeans on over the bathing suit and one of those long shapeless man's shirts that I wore all the time anyway. I almost carried my beach bag with me, but then I realized how feminine that would look. Instead, I rolled up a towel and put it under my arm, the way the guys did when they went to the beach.

It was a hot, sunny day. The bus seemed to take forever to get to its destination. By the time it arrived, I was so nervous that I wasn't sure I'd be able to go through with it. I decided to take one step at a time. I walked along the sandy beach with a crowd of other people. After looking carefully around to make sure there was no one there who knew me, I spread my towel out on the sand.

I glanced around again, feeling a little paranoid and wanting to make certain that no one would recognize me. Then I slipped out of the jeans. I stood there in my stuffed Speedo, wondering if anybody had noticed me. At last, I took the final step and removed the shirt. Nobody seemed to give me a second look.

I lowered myself onto the towel and braced my body back onto my elbows. The sun felt nice and warm against my naked chest. Not even a breeze disturbed the still air. Boy, did this feel wonderful. Not only were my bare tits exposed to the elements, they were exposed to the sight of anyone who cared to look. My nipples were as hard as diamonds. I hadn't even imagined how exciting it would turn out to be.

That first time, I just contented myself with lying there on the towel. When I went back to the beach the following day, I got a little bolder. After removing my shirt and jeans, I walked along the edge of the surf for a mile or more, feeling the ocean breeze caressing my bare nipples and exposing myself to hundreds of unsuspecting bathers.

Occasionally, someone walking past me would glance in my direction. Maybe his eyes would glide casually over my body, not even stopping to linger at my erect little pink nipples. For me, the feeling was electrifying. It was as if he were actually touching me, stroking the sensitive tissues. I could feel myself getting wet inside the Speedo.

That summer, I went to the beach as often as I could, at least two or three times a week, sometimes every day. On a few occasions, I took off my shirt while riding to or from the beach. Sitting there bare-breasted in the middle of the crowded bus was even more daring, and that made it more exciting. When I got home from my topless excursions, I would head straight for my bedroom and rub my nipples and my clitoris until I came again and again.

After that, I kept my hair cut short and took every possible opportunity to pass myself off as a boy. Even in college, I would take a bus to the next town and walk shirtless in the streets on warm days. Sometimes I'd go into a coffee shop with a sign on the door that said, NO SHIRT, NO SHOES, NO SERVICE. I'd put the shirt on, but leave it totally unbuttoned so my nipples would show. Nobody ever caught on.

Eventually, I met Darrel. After a whirlwind romance, we got married. He never complained about my shape, but I sensed that he wished I was more feminine-looking. Deep down I knew a day would come when he'd want me to do something about it. I was right.

First, he asked me to let my hair grow. Then he started talking about getting me a boob job. I resisted for as long as I could, saying I was worried about all the trouble women were having with implants. I couldn't tell him the truth. How could I say I didn't want a boob job because I liked passing myself off as a boy and showing my naked nipples to the world?

He surprised me on my birthday with a certificate for a visit to a plastic surgeon. I guess it was kind of a dirty trick. After all, how could I refuse a birthday present? The doctor talked about the relative safety of saline implants instead of silicon ones. That convinced Darrel. I didn't really feel I had any choice but to go along with it.

Now I have these big boobs that everyone likes to look at. Darrel certainly enjoys playing with them. For a long time after the operation, I had no sensation at all in my nipples. After a while, though, that came back.

Darrel likes paying a lot of attention to them, stroking and licking and sucking. I must admit it feels good. Too bad that my days of going topless in a Speedo bathing suit are over, though. I sure do miss the thrill I got from being half-naked in public, while passing myself off as a boy. There was something about it that I'll never be able to describe to Darrel or anyone else. Maybe your readers will understand.

NINE
Watching My Own Mate

*I*n Shakespeare's *Othello*, Iago describes jealousy as a green-eyed monster that mocks the meat it feeds on. That monster destroys Othello and has since destroyed many other men and women. Most cannot resist it, however, even when they know its devastating effects.

Some psychologists have suggested that jealousy is one of the innate emotions with which we are born. The way married people battle over real or imagined encounters with others—even those that occurred before the marriage—seems to support the innate emotion theory. There are some, however, who have so overcome the green-eyed monster that they manage to derive erotic excitement from their mates' extramarital sexual contacts.

Elizabeth, who tells her story in this chapter, finds herself becoming highly aroused at recollections of seeing her husband making love to her cousin. Al, who planned to catch his wife with her lover and fully expected to become violent as a result, discovered that watching them couple was an aphrodisiac that renewed his marriage and reinvigorated his sexual interest. It is ironic, perhaps, that although both receive erotic satisfaction from seeing their partners with others, neither is willing to confess the unspoken desire to see more of the same, though their partners probably would be most willing to oblige.

Husband and Cousin

*E*lizabeth, twenty-eight, is employed as a legal secretary. She stands right around five feet tall and tips the scale at one hundred thirty pounds. Her rounded figure is attractive in a renaissance sort of way. Her moon face is surrounded by a mass of curly red hair. Freckles are sprinkled across the bridge of her nose and spattered over her plump cheeks. Her brown eyes flash as she tells us about her husband and her cousin.

When I first moved to this city, I didn't know a soul except my cousin Krystal, and I hardly knew her. Her mother and my mother are sisters, but they live at opposite ends of the country and haven't spoken to each other for years. At first, I was hesitant about contacting her. But I never really knew what it was that had come between our mothers, and I didn't really see any reason why it should be an issue between us. So when I knew I was coming here, I called her to ask for advice.

To my surprise, she seemed glad to hear from me. "This is a big, unfriendly city," she said. "It's going to take you a while to find your way around. Until you do, I insist that you stay with me." Her former roommate had just moved out, and she needed someone to share the rent. I had some meager savings that I was planning to live on while looking for a job. No doubt it would be to our mutual benefit to join forces.

I hadn't seen Krystal since we were kids and wasn't sure I'd recognize her. When she came to the door of her apartment, though, I knew her at once. She looks a lot different than me. She's tall and slender, while I'm kind of short and chunky. But the red hair and freckles are like a family trademark, and hers are just like mine. We embraced and she pulled me inside.

She said, "Now, tell me all about yourself." Then she proceeded to talk a blue streak, without giving me a chance to get a single word in edgewise. She described her social life in great detail. She was dating lots and lots of guys, all on a casual basis, and promised to introduce me to some of them. She kept saying that life in the city was more fun than I could even imagine and that I was going to love it there.

She was working as an administrator in a large law office. Since I had received training as a legal secretary at a business college back home, she thought she could get me a job there. Finally, when she ran out of things to say about herself, she repeated her opening line, "Now, tell me all about you." Before I could answer, she flew into the kitchen to start a pot of coffee.

I soon found this to be Krystal's style. She was very interested in herself and not much else. Jokingly, she used to say, "Well, that's enough about me. Let's talk about you. What do you think of me?" She was fun, though, and really good-natured.

She did succeed in getting me that job. Based upon what I learned about unemployment in this town, I don't know if I could have survived here without her help. We both worked hard all week and lived for the weekends. They were never boring around Krystal. She seemed to know a thousand different people, mostly men. There were always crowds dropping in and out of the apartment to laugh and talk and socialize. I got to know quite a few of them.

My favorite was James, one of her many boyfriends. He was an attorney, who worked for a firm with offices in the same building as the lawyers we worked for. He was bright and very handsome. I found myself rather attracted to him. I never would have dreamed of making a play for him, because I regarded him as Krystal's property, even though she told me I was welcome to him. She said that even though he was the best lay in town, she'd gladly give him up if I was the least bit interested.

Krystal was very frank about her sexuality. When we were alone together, she thought nothing of walking around totally nude. She was so explicit about the relationships she had with her male friends that I was embarrassed at first. After a time, I got used to it. I even started walking around naked, myself, something I had never done at home.

We would sit together on the living room couch wearing nothing at all. Krystal would be doing her nails and telling me all about the man she had slept with the night before. She used words that I wasn't used to hearing, but, somehow, coming from her, it didn't seem dirty. She especially liked talking about James.

"That man can eat pussy like no one else," she'd say. "He gets his tongue all the way inside and just rolls it around until I'm ready to melt. Then he starts licking me up and down like a great big lollipop until I blow my cookies. You ought to see the dick on him. Bigger than anything I ever saw. Really huge. He certainly knows what to do with it, too.

"He's different from most guys. All they're interested in is getting their own nuts off. Not James. He'll fuck you until you come hundred times if you let him. He says his greatest pleasure is getting a woman off. Well, I guess they all say that. But he really means it."

All her talk about James and his sexual ability made me more interested in him than ever. Sometimes, at night, when I was alone in my bed, I'd fantasize about him and rub myself to orgasm. As I came, I'd imagine him licking me the way Krystal described it, or I'd think of his big penis entering me. At that point, my fingers were my only sex partners. In spite of the introductions my cousin made, I just hadn't found any-one I really wanted to go to bed with.

One day at work, I felt sort of feverish and thought I might be coming down with something. So I decided to go home early. After clearing it with my supervisor, I told Krystal and left. I went straight home, got into bed, and fell asleep right away.

A few hours later, I was awakened by sounds in the living room. My bedroom door was partially open. By leaning out of the bed, I could see Krystal sitting on the couch. I was about to call out a greeting when I realized that she wasn't alone. James was with her. He had one arm around her shoulders. His other hand was fiddling with the buttons on the front of her blouse.

I held my breath as I watched him undress her. Off came the blouse and bra, and out came her breasts. Immediately, he began stroking and petting them. I could hear her moaning softly and I could see her reaching for his crotch. In a moment, his penis was protruding from his open fly. She held it lovingly in her hand and started rubbing it lightly up and down. I saw it getting stiffer and harder. It grew longer and thicker, until I realized that Krystal had been telling the truth when she said he was absolutely huge.

For a moment, I felt a little guilty about invading their privacy by peeking at them. I thought of getting up and closing my door, but that would let them know that I had been watching. I thought of turning around and trying to go back to sleep, but, to tell you the truth, I couldn't tear my eyes off them. Krystal's descriptions had got me wondering and fantasizing about James and his sexual technique. Now I was getting to see it firsthand.

After a few minutes, they were both naked. His body was firm and strong. The hair on his chest was an arousing sight. It was dark and thick, narrowing down to a vertical band that went all the way to his waist, where it flared out to form a dark curly triangle. Below it, I could see his erection, standing hard and tall. He was the most exciting man I ever saw.

I had seen my cousin without her clothes on dozens of times, but she looked sexier now that her body was next to his. The red hair of her pubes stood out like a flame against the soft whiteness of her skin. Her pink nipples were erect and seemed to be crying for his attention.

Slowly, he placed his hands on her breasts and pushed her back against the cushions of the couch. She spread her legs open, throwing one of them over the back of the couch. Although I had seen her naked, I never had an opportunity like this to look right into her open vulva. It was sex itself.

He sat there staring at it for a moment and then eased himself forward. I could see him kissing the rosy lips that surrounded her opening before dabbing at them with the tip of his tongue. Slowly, thoroughly, he lapped at every part of her open vagina, each movement of his mouth bringing a soft moan from her throat.

He stiffened his tongue and drove it inside, undulating his head back and forth to mimic the movements of intercourse. It was just the way she had described it. He seemed to be rolling his tongue around inside her. She did seem ready to melt. When I saw her body beginning to wriggle, I wondered if I was actually going to witness her having an orgasm. A moment later, I was sure of it. Her hips thrashed wildly, but his mouth rode her all the way, never leaving her vagina for an instant. She seemed to rise up off the couch as her climax lifted her higher and higher.

I closed my eyes and imagined it was me that he was eating. Oh, it felt so good. How I envied her. When I opened my eyes again, he was mounting her. I was just in time to see his huge penis sliding into her wet and open vagina.

Their groins moved as one, coming together and then pulling apart as though choreographed. What a sight! I'm sure I saw her have five or six climaxes before he finally announced with a grunt that he was achieving his completion inside her. They continued moving together for a time before settling down to lie still in each other's arms, breathing heavily. They whispered for a while, Then he got up, dressed, and left. I stayed awake the rest of the night, replaying what I had seen, as I fingered myself to one orgasm after another.

After that, I had several other opportunities to see the two of them making love. I wasn't jealous of my cousin in a hostile way. I certainly envied the pleasure that she received from James, though. I longed to tell her I had been watching and to ask her about what she felt while making love to him, but I couldn't let her know that I had been peeking.

Watching them became the erotic highlight of my life. I had seen a couple of porno movies at parties, but nothing had ever been as exciting as actually witnessing Krystal and James having sex, live and in person. I didn't know how I would ever be able to find a man of my own after seeing the likes of James.

One day Krystal asked me why I didn't go out with men. I had to confess that the only man I was attracted to was already taken. She grinned and asked me to tell her about it, obviously expecting to hear a tale of exotic romance. After hesitating for a moment, I told her that I had a crush on James. To my dismay, she burst out laughing.

"Well, take him, then," she said. "As long as you don't mind knowing that he's given me some of the best fucking I've ever had. What the hell, there are lots of other men out there. He doesn't mean anything special to me. Go ahead, he's yours."

"That's very generous of you," I said. "But don't you think he might have something to say about it?"

She just laughed. "Why don't you leave that to me?" she said.

I don't know what Krystal had to do with it or how she arranged it, but about a week later, James asked me out to dinner. As we chatted, it turned out that we had a lot in common. I really enjoyed his company. I knew I would enjoy having sex with him, because all I could think about were the things I had seen him doing with Krystal. When he invited me back to his place for a drink, I jumped at the chance.

I guess I was the easiest make of his life. We hadn't taken two sips of our drinks before we were naked and in each other's arms. He treated me to that special oral sex that he was so good at, and then we had the longest most intense intercourse of my life. Through it all, I pictured him doing the same things to Krystal. Instead of making me jealous, it turned me on, raising me to places even higher than he was taking me to. Imagining him going down on Krystal and slipping his penis into her was a tool that brought me to crashing orgasm again and again.

A few months after that first date, I moved in with James. Soon after that, we were married. Our life has been absolutely blissful since then. We make passionate love every night, and every time we do it, I visualize him with my cousin. It's gotten to the point where I don't think I can have orgasms without picturing the two of them. Sometimes I imagine the three of us all in one bed, with me just sitting back and watching while he does all those wonderful things to her.

I've never told him, though. I guess, somewhere inside, I'm afraid that if he knew how turned on it makes me to think of him having sex with another woman, he would take that as a kind of license to fool around. Even though I love imagining it, I don't think I could stand it if I found out he was actually cheating on me. It would be so easy for him with Krystal, too, because of her casual attitude about sex. So this secret of mine is going to remain forever unspoken.

Attic

$\mathcal{A}$ l is dark-haired and dark-eyed, with olive skin and two perfect rows of shining white teeth. He is thirty years old, and a little over six feet tall, with broad shoulders and a trim waist. Along with his good looks goes a friendly personality that makes him easy to talk to. He looks like an athlete, but he isn't. He is self-employed as a painting contractor and says he doesn't believe in working too hard.

I don't know how it happened, but after just a few years of marriage, I found myself losing sexual interest in my wife. It wasn't her. She's a real knockout. Tall and shapely, with long dark curly hair and the bluest eyes you ever saw. She's got a dynamite pair of legs and her tits—well, those tits are what first attracted me to her. Big and round, without any help from a plastic surgeon. Best of all, she's got a sexual appetite that knows no bounds.

When we first got married, we used to fuck like bunnies. A couple of times a night, and in the morning, too. On weekends, we'd sometimes spend the whole day going from one fuck to another—in bed, on the living room floor, on the kitchen counter, in the shower, anyplace you can think of. Maybe it was just a case of too much of a good thing. Anyway, after a while, I just started slowing down and losing interest.

She'd nudge me in bed at night and I'd roll over and grudgingly put one to her. Then I'd turn around and go right to sleep. In the morning, I'd be sure to get up before she was awake so she wouldn't ask for another one. I started going to sleep earlier and earlier so there wouldn't be any chance for sex at nighttime, either. Before you knew it, we practically stopped fucking altogether. I knew that Sherry had her needs, but I just didn't give a shit. I wasn't interested. I just wasn't in the mood. Ever.

So it shouldn't have come as a surprise—and maybe it didn't—when I started suspecting her of having an affair. She'd be on the phone and then hang up the second I came into the room. Or I'd call her at work and they'd tell me she went home early, but when I called her at home the phone would just ring and ring.

One night, I went to bed early and was pretending to be asleep so I wouldn't have to get it up, when the phone rang. She was in the living room at the time, but before she answered it, she took the trouble to close the bedroom door. That really tipped me off. Quiet as I could, I got out of bed and crept to the door, pressing my ear against it. She was talking in a low voice, but I could hear her anyway.

She mentioned the name Josh a few times. I didn't know anybody by that name and had no idea who it was. It was obvious that she was arranging to meet him the next day. She said, "Yes, I'll be home around two o'clock. Can you get here then?" He must have said he could, because she said, "Okay, I can't wait," and then hung up.

Later, when she came into the bedroom, I acted like nothing had happened. I just lay there breathing deep and making believe I was asleep. I had already hatched my plan. After she left for work, I would go up to the attic and drill a little peephole so I could see into the bedroom. I'd wait until two o'clock when she met her lover. I'd spy on them through the hole until I had the goods on them. Then I'd rush into the bedroom and catch them right in the act. I'd beat the shit out of him and I'd beat the living daylights out of her, too. I wasn't even that upset. In fact, I was kind of excited about the idea of busting them.

The next day, when I heard her come into the house a little after one-thirty, I got ready to put my plan into action. I hunkered down on the attic floor with my eye pressed to the hole I had drilled. I could see her getting ready for her little rendezvous.

She took off all her clothes and doused herself with perfume. Then she put on a sexy lace bra and panties set. I recognized it. In fact, I had bought it for her a couple of years earlier. I don't ever remember her wearing it for me. Now the bitch was putting it on for this total stranger.

I must admit she looked good in it. Her big tits overflowed the cups of that pink bra just enough to be enticing. I could almost see her round nipples through the lace. The dark triangle of hair around her pussy showed right through the material of the panties. She's got a real fur muff down there, which she keeps untrimmed. There was a time that really turned me on. As I lay on the attic floor, weird as it seemed, I found it turning me on again. My cock was even getting a little hard. Just as I started to wonder if she was going to wear anything else, she took a sheer pink robe from her closet and slipped it on over the sexy underwear. Man, she looked good. It made me think of the days when our lives were filled with sex.

I heard a knock at the front door. She disappeared from my view as she went to answer it. For a moment I worried that, the way she looked, they might not make it back to the bedroom. They might just end up doing it on the living room floor like she and I had done so many times. I cursed myself for not thinking of that and drilling a few more peepholes so I could see her wherever she went. A minute later, she came back into the bedroom, leading a man by the hand. He wasn't much to look at—short and kind of skinny.

As soon as they were in the room, they started kissing. I could see her lips press against his and I could imagine her tongue snaking down his throat in that hungry, horny way she has of communicating her desire. He was groaning, and his hands were starting to roam over her body. When he cupped her tits through the robe and bra, I saw her body move in tight against his, her pussy grinding his crotch.

I couldn't believe this was really happening. Here I was hiding in the attic watching as my wife gave it to this guy I never saw or heard of before. How far should I let it go before I busted in on them? I already had enough reason to get down there and start kicking some ass.

While I thought about it, she wriggled out of the robe and stepped back so he could look at her in the bra and panties. I could see that the sight affected him, because the front of his pants was starting to make like a tent. Right before my eyes, she dropped to her knees before him and opened his zipper. Then she unbuckled his belt and yanked his pants and drawers down around his ankles, freeing his cock. It was big and stiff. Oh, God, she was going to give him a blowjob.

I watched, horrified, as she took his dick in her mouth and started sucking on it. The minute her red lips closed around it, he started to moan. His eyes were closed and his hips were swaying back and forth as he fucked my wife's mouth. She looked like she was enjoying it as much as him. Her eyes were closed tight and her cheeks were puffing in and out as she sucked on his prick. Her hands reached up to play with his balls and to stroke the base of his cock while she ate him.

I thought of the days when she used to do stuff like that to me. I could remember just how it felt and I could imagine what this guy Josh was feeling. In my memory, I was experiencing that free sensation I used to get when I just let it go and pumped my cum down her swallowing throat. I was hoping that he wouldn't come in her mouth. In a weird way, I was also hoping that he would. For some really strange reason, I wanted to see it.

It was like he read my mind. "I'm going to come," he moaned. "I'm going to let it fly."

I was kind of disappointed when she pulled away from him and grabbed his cock with her hand and started squeezing it. "No," she whispered. "Don't come yet. I want to feel you fuck me."

She threw herself back on the bed and spread her legs wide apart. In the blink of an eye, he was out of his pants and shoes and had drawn his shirt off over his head. He reached down and took hold of her pink panties, tearing them right off her body. I could see the lips of her pussy, all red and open, waiting for his cock the way they used to wait for mine.

I knew it was time for me to run down there and kick open the door before he got his cock into her. But I couldn't move. I was actually enjoying the sight of my wife and this guy making it together. I didn't want to do anything to stop it. First, I wanted to see his cock go into her. I wanted to see her legs wrap around his waist. Then I could break them up.

I watched in helpless fascination as he undid the clasp at the front of her bra and pulled it away from her tits. They were round and full, with dark nipples, hardened with desire. He bent over her and started sucking on them, making loud noises. While he licked her nipples, she reached for his cock and guided it toward her waiting pussy. It was about to enter her.

I was about to see this guy fuck my wife. I was fastened to the spot, unable to move a muscle. My own cock was so hard it was aching. I couldn't remember the last time I felt such excitement.

With a quick thrust, he drove his hard-on deep inside Sherry's belly, bringing a gasp of delight from her throat. "Oh, yeah," she moaned. "Fuck me. Fuck me deep."

I watched his ass bobbing up and down as he drove his cock in and out of her. I never would have believed that I would find the sight of another man fucking my wife to be so exciting. I actually had to tighten all the muscles of my ass to keep myself from coming in my pants.

He kept fucking her and fucking her. She kept crying out in pleasure as she wrapped her legs and arms around him, drawing him so tight against her that their bodies merged into one tangled mass of erotic flesh. "Oh, I'm going to come," I heard her shout. "I want to feel you come in me. Fill my pussy with your cum."

The obscenities that were spewing from her mouth went straight to my nuts. I couldn't hold it back anymore. I could feel my cock rising and swelling and then, boom, letting go, pumping hot juice into my pants as I came in time with my wife and her lover on the bed in the room below me. It was the best come I ever had in my life.

When it was over, I knew I couldn't do anything to spoil the scene taking place in my bedroom. My wife had just given me the hottest sex I had in a very long time by fucking a stranger while I watched. I found myself wishing they would do it again. After a few minutes, Josh got up and put his clothes back on. Sherry was still lying there with her legs spread. He dropped to his knees at the foot of the bed and planted a loud smacking kiss on her wet pussy before leaving the room and the house.

After he was gone, she petted her pussy with her hand for a while and then got up and began straightening out the room. I just stayed in the attic, as quiet as I could be. After a while, she went into the shower, and I took the opportunity to slip out of the house.

When I came in the door later that evening, Sherry acted as if nothing had happened. So did I, except that, for the first time in more than a year, I wanted to fuck her. She was trying to get dinner on the table when I started grabbing her ass and feeling her tits. She giggled. "Hey, Al," she said. "What's gotten into you?"

"Never mind what's gotten into me," I answered. "I want to get into you. Right here."

Sherry lifted her skirt and bent over the kitchen table. She didn't have any panties on and was pointing her naked ass at me. I couldn't help thinking that another man had shot a load into her pussy just a few hours earlier. "Go ahead," she whispered in a husky voice. "Fuck me fast and hard, the way you used to."

I dropped my pants and stuck it in her, thrusting in and

out with a series of quick strokes. All the while, my head was filled with the image of her sucking Josh's cock and then lying on her back while he shoved it into her pussy like I was doing now. Within seconds, I came, pumping my load into her waiting body. When I was done, she giggled again.

"I like it like that," she said. "We need to do it more. Whatever it is that led you to this, I like it."

For a moment, I thought of telling her what I had seen. But I was embarrassed. After all, how could I let her know that I had been spying on her. Worst of all, how could I admit that I knew she was fucking another guy and it was all right with me. More than all right. That I enjoyed it. That's not a very manly thing to feel and not a very romantic thing to tell your wife. So I just shrugged it off. "I don't know," I said. "But I like it, too."

I was hoping that I would get a chance to see her with Josh again. She didn't let me down. In fact, it turns out he's just one of several guys she's been fucking on the side. I've sort of figured out the schedule. I try to be in my attic hideaway whenever she's got a hot date cooking. I've drilled a few more peepholes, so I can see her wherever she does it. Then, after spending an hour or so watching her fuck another man, I get so hot and horny that we end up having great sex again, just like we used to.

I've decided I won't ever tell her. I'll just keep this little secret to myself. Why screw up a good thing?

TEN

Same Gender

The Old Testament prohibits men from lying with other men as they would with women, calling the practice an "abomination." (Leviticus 20:13). Recently, fundamentalists have used this passage to justify their campaign against equal rights for homosexuals. Some have even suggested that AIDS is a heavenly punishment for violation of the biblical exhortation.

We find it interesting that the same fundamentalists generally do not refrain from eating pork, or recommend the death penalty for people who disrespect their parents. Both of these proscriptions are also found in the Old Testament. In addition, since female homosexuals have a lower incidence of AIDS than most other groups, we wonder why the fundamentalists do not see this as a heavenly reward.

In spite of society's increasingly live-and-let-live sexual attitude, male homosexuals face discrimination and sometimes even violence as a result of their sexual preference. Perhaps this explains why Elroy, who tells his story in this chapter, associates his homosexual fantasy with shame and embarrassment. On the other hand, Frances, who actually is involved in an extramarital lesbianic affair, keeps it secret for another reason. She longs for a world in which her sexual interest in another woman would be understood and tolerated, and keeps her desire unspoken only because she believes that her husband would not approve.

Imaginary Threesome

$\mathcal{E}$lroy, a car salesman, is in his late forties and stands about six-foot-three. His lanky body is a little on the awkward side, as though he never quite knows what to do with it. His chocolate-colored hands are constantly fidgeting with each other, his fingers twining and intertwining. His eyes, like his hair, are black, but without any real luster. He has a thin wisp of a moustache, neatly trimmed but sparse. When he speaks, his lips seem to struggle to form the words before any sound comes out.

I wish I could tell my wife about this fantasy of mine, but I don't think I'll ever be able to do that. I wouldn't want Rheta to lose all respect for me. I just know she would if she heard about it.

It started about a year ago. We were at a party, having a pretty good time, drinking wine, smoking a little weed. I must have drank too much, because I ended up passing out in a chair. Don't know how long I was passed out, but gradually I became aware of the party still going on around me. I kept my eyes closed for a few minutes, trying to get orientated.

I heard people laughing, you know, and the tinkle of glasses and stuff. So I opened my eyes slowly and looked around a little. The chair I was in was facing a sofa. There, sitting on it was my wife and this guy, Jerome. I'd seen him around some, but I didn't really know him. I didn't think

Rheta knew him, either. Apparently she did. In fact, she seemed to know him real well.

They were sitting side by side, and her hand was in his lap. The zipper of his pants was open, and his cock was sticking straight up, big and hard. I tell you, it looked like a circumcised baseball bat. My wife's hand was wrapped around it, slowly stroking it up and down.

I knew I should be pissed off. I guess I was a little, but mainly I found the sight very arousing. He had the biggest cock I ever saw. Watching it jump and twitch in her hand was more exciting than I would have expected it to be. They were so wrapped up in each other that they didn't notice that I was awake and watching. I just kept my mouth shut. I was hoping that she'd keep doing it until he came. I wanted to see that.

It looked like he was getting ready to. His dick swelled up even bigger as my wife's hand movements got faster. He started gasping for breath. I figured it was going to be a real shower. Then he glanced over at me and muttered, "Oh, shit." I saw his cock go limp all of a sudden. He got up without a word, zipped his pants, and darted out of the room.

Rheta just stared at me for a moment. Then her face got all screwed up and she started to cry. "Oh, Elroy," she wailed. "I don't know what came over me. Oh, I'm so sorry. Oh, baby, I'm so sorry."

We were beginning to attract some attention from the other people at the party, so I just said, real cold, "Get our things. We're leaving."

Docile as a lamb, she went into the bedroom for her coat and mine. When she came out, her face was wet with tears. By the time we got to the car, she was wailing again, copping all kinds of a plea. "Oh, baby, I don't know what came over me. I was just so drunk. I got carried away. Oh, God, how can I make this up to you? I'll do anything you want. I'll give you anything you want. Anything. Baby, I'm sooo sorry."

I acted like I was real angry, but to tell the truth, I kept picturing his giant cock in her hand, and the picture was giving me a hard-on. "I ought to kill you," I said. "And maybe I will. But for now, you just suck me off while I drive us home. Then, we'll see."

She did as I had ordered, opening my pants and taking my cock in her mouth while I drove. I came within seconds and made her swallow every drop of it. For the rest of the drive, I was absolutely silent. When we got home, I made her sleep on the floor next to the bed.

For a week or so after that, I didn't talk to her much. She thought I was seething with anger and did her best to soften me up. She'd cook my favorite foods and wait on me hand and foot. Sometimes, she'd drop her pants and bend over with her rear pointing out at me, inviting me to stick it in her for a fast fuck. I took advantage of every offer, but showed no emotion. Truth is, each time I'd slide my cock into her, I'd picture Jerome's big sticker.

After a while, I decided to let her off the hook. I said, "Remember, you said you'd do anything to make up to me for that night with Jerome? Okay, I've decided what I want."

"Anything, baby," she said. "Just forgive me."

"Okay," I answered in an authoritative voice. "I want you to go to the store and buy a strap-on dildo. You're going to do this all by yourself, now. Then I want you to come back here and fuck me in the ass with it." She looked relieved. "First, you'll have to lick my asshole inside and out to get it lubricated."

She still looked relieved. "Sure, baby," she said. "Anything you say. I'll go right now if you want me to."

"Tomorrow will be time enough," I said. "You'd just better have it here by the time I get home from work."

The next day, I had the shakes all day long. All I could think about was Rheta's promise. I tell you, my ass was tingling. I just couldn't wait to get home. When I did, she was there for me, practically naked. She had on a skimpy little bed-jacket that kept opening up to show her titties. Rheta has giant titties. I could also see the dark curly patch of hair around her pussy. Sticking out from the hairy tangle was a stiff rubber cock.

It was so big that it made me sorry I had asked her to fuck me with it. I couldn't imagine how I was going to be able to take it up my ass. But the thought of it really turned me on. I couldn't help comparing it to the size of Jerome's big dick. Through my haze, I heard my Rheta talking. "I've got it, baby," she whispered. "Just like you wanted. I'm going to fuck you with it all night, if you want. I'm going to give it to you any way you like, over and over again. And I'm ready to start right now."

With that, she stepped up and began opening my pants. I just stood there, letting her do the work. Pretty soon, I was completely naked and she was running her hands over my chest, playing with my nipples, and then reaching down to take my cock and balls into both her hands. She stroked them so softly that I was hard as a rock within seconds. I started handling her pussy and found her to be wetter than ever. She was enjoying this penance that I had imposed on her.

She fell to her knees and started licking my nuts, flattening her tongue out good and wide and painting broad strokes over my scrotum. Then she began flicking at the base of my cock with just the tip of her tongue. Involuntarily, I sighed. Taking that as a kind of signal, I guess, she started working her way toward the back, lapping up the crease between my ass cheeks, getting closer and closer to my asshole. I heard groaning and realized that it was me. Her tongue was working circles around the tight hole now, wetting it and greasing it, like she was getting it ready for an entry.

In my mind, I was seeing a picture of Jerome's cock in her hand. Somehow, that changed to a picture of Jerome's cock in my hand. Then, as she worked one of her fingers into my asshole, I pictured Jerome's cock going in me there. I leaned over to let Rheta have a clear shot and I felt her pressing the tip of the strap-on dildo against my opening.

God, it felt too good to describe. She worked it in slowly,

and there was plenty of pain, but it still felt terrific. Inch after inch penetrated my ass, and the whole time I kept picturing Jerome's baseball bat driving into me. I've always been straight. Never had any contact or interest in another man, but this was the most exciting picture I can ever remember.

When she had the dildo all the way in, she started fucking me, by moving her hips back and forth. My cock was hard as a rock and sticking straight out in front of me. She reached around me and grabbed it and started jerking it up and down to match the rhythm of the rubber dick in my ass. Good thing she did, because I came within seconds. I wouldn't have wanted her to know it was the dildo that got me off. That and the picture of Jerome's prick up my ass.

We spent the rest of the night having sex, with her wearing that dildo like it was her own cock and fucking me with it in various positions. I just couldn't seem to get enough. Every time I thought I was totally spent, my dick would start getting hard again, and I'd demand another one. Sometimes, I took it on my hands and knees. Sometimes, I'd lie on my back with my legs in the air like a woman. Sometimes, I'd be on my side, and she'd give it to me spoon-fashion. By morning, I was so exhausted that I had to call in sick to work.

I spent the day in bed, nursing my sore ass and dozing off. When I was awake, I had fantasies of being fucked by Jerome. When I slept, I dreamed about it. I've had this fantasy ever since. It's really my favorite. I'm lying in a hammock in the backyard when Rheta tells me she's going out for a while. Then, just before leaving, she says, "Jerome's coming over. I told him he could do whatever he wanted to you while I'm gone."

I fall asleep in the hammock, wearing only a brief pair of shorts. When I wake up, there are hands on me, feeling my cock through the shorts. I keep my eyes closed for another moment and the hands begin pulling down the shorts. My cock is throbbing and twitching all over the place.

I open my eyes just in time to see Jerome kneeling down beside the hammock and leaning over to breathe his hot breath on my cock. Then he takes it into his mouth and starts licking and sucking on it. It feels so good to be getting a blowjob in the middle of the afternoon in my backyard that, for the moment, I forget who's doing the sucking. Then I remember and my cock begins to jump. I want to come in his mouth and I just do. My belly churns as I pump my load down his throat, and he swallows it all gladly.

When I'm done, he stands up and takes off his pants. He's wearing white jockeys, and I can see the huge bulge made by his swollen cock. "Take these off me," he orders. I do it, and his hard-on springs into view. "Roll over," he commands. "I'm going to stick this thing right up your ass."

I feel weak at the thought of what's about to happen. But I manage to do as I'm told, rolling over and lifting my ass in the air for him. He doesn't lick it to grease it up, the way Rheta did. He just pushes his cock against it and shoves. At first, it hurts like holy hell, but he doesn't care. He just drives on. Somehow, the pain begins to turn into pleasure and then into positive joy, as that giant hunk of meat presses deeper and deeper into me.

He fucks me like that until I'm about to come again, when I hear the car pulling into the driveway. It's Rheta, back home. I get nervous. I'm having too good a time and I don't want her to know it. I'm thinking of jumping up out of the hammock, but it's too late. She's there, standing beside it, watching Jerome's dick sliding in and out my ass.

She lifts her skirt and pulls her panties to one side, showing me and Jerome her bright pink pussy. Then she starts rubbing it. At the sight of her watching and showing us her stuff, I explode. Big spurts of cum shoot from my cock as Jerome's dick penetrates as far as it can go. Suddenly, Rheta creeps under the hammock and starts licking my cock from below, while Jerome keeps fucking my ass.

At last my cock gets soft, and I struggle to catch my breath. Jerome takes his dick out of me and stands there with it stiff and swaying in the breeze. Rheta stands up and puts one foot on a chair, opening her pussy wide for us to see. Then she reaches out and takes Jerome's cock in her hand and pulls him toward her. She guides the huge organ into her opening and begins hollering as he drives it all the way in. I feel myself getting hard again as I watch the man who just fucked my ass now fucking my wife. I don't feel any jealousy or anger, just excitement. I want to see her come. I want to see him come in her.

They fuck that way for a long time, with me watching and stroking my own cock. Finally, she starts to breathe hoarsely and heavily and begins to shout. "Oh, Elroy," she wails. "I'm going to come. Oh, yes, I'm almost there. Oooohhhh."

I recognize the sounds she makes as she has an orgasm. I see Jerome's rhythm change and the muscles of his ass go all tense. I know that he's about to come, too. I get up out of the hammock and press my stiff cock between the cheeks of his ass while he pumps his load into my wife's pussy. They keep fucking as I enter him. I fuck him until I shoot my load inside Jerome's asshole.

Then I fall to my knees and start eating Rheta's pussy, getting off on the taste of the mixture of her juices and his cum dribbling out of her. Even while I'm doing it, my cock gets hard again, as I think about the wonderful threesome that we're going to have.

Now it's become almost impossible for me to have sex with Rheta without picturing this little scenario, or some variation on it. You can understand why I'll never be able to tell her. Too bad, though, because I have a feeling that if I did, she'd be willing.

Afternoon Delight

*F*rances, thirty-seven, describes herself as a part-time freelance writer and part-time housewife. She is of medium height and a little thick around the middle. Her large bosom is a bit droopy. Her long blond hair, worn in an artsy French braid, frames her moon-shaped face. Her light brown eyes are surrounded by metal-rimmed glasses. When we meet with her, her face wears a rosy flush and she seems a little breathless.

I've decided to tell you guys everything, even though I don't know you at all. Maybe that's why. Besides, talking about it might help relieve me of this burden I've been carrying for so long. You see, I'm happily married, but I just got back from spending an afternoon with my lover.

You don't look at all shocked. Well, I guess you hear that sort of thing from married women all the time. How about if I tell you that my lover's name is Marsha and that she's a woman? What, still not shocked? Or do you just keep a straight face for professional reasons? Well, anyway, let me tell you all about it.

Marsha and I grew up on the same street in our little hometown. It's just a coincidence that we both live in this city now. At least I think it is. Anyway, even though Marsha is four years older than I, we've been the best of friends since I was ten years old. I know it's kind of strange for a fourteen-year-old to hang out with a ten-year-old, but as I look back on it now, I realize that it was probably because Marsha was

so different from the other girls her age. They were all interested in boys. Marsha wasn't. She was interested in girls.

I didn't know that then, of course. It seemed perfectly
natural for her to spend time with me. We were crazy about
each other. We did everything together, from riding our bikes
in the country to dressing up and going to Friday-night con-
certs at the high school auditorium.

It wasn't until I finished high school that I realized Marsha
was not like the other girls I knew. She had become an artist
by then and had her own apartment, which she also used as
a studio. She invited me over to celebrate my graduation and
my eighteenth birthday, which came at just about the same
time. In our state, it was legal for eighteen-year-olds to drink,
so she made some punch. It tasted like lemonade, but had
just a little vodka in it. It was so mild that I probably would
have needed ten gallons of it to get drunk, but I felt terribly
adult just knowing there was alcohol in it.

At some point, we were sitting together on a sofa, and
Marsha's arm was around my shoulders. It was a nice sensation. I always felt safe and warm around her. I was comfortable and relaxed. When she kissed me, it seemed perfectly
natural for me to kiss back. At first, it was just a light brushing
of the lips. In seconds it grew into a more passionate kiss.
When I felt her tongue entering my mouth, I got all tingly
inside. Then her hands were on my breasts and, suddenly, I
was all confused.

I had been out with a few boys and had done some kissing
in the backseats of their cars. A few of them had tried feeling
me up, but I always put a stop to it after a minute or two. I
couldn't deny that it felt good, but I had been brought up to
believe that it was wrong, and I really did believe that.

Somehow, though, this was different. For one thing, Marsha was a girl. Girls could do things together that they
couldn't do with boys. Like going into the same dressing
room in the department store, or seeing each other naked in
the locker room at the swimming pool. For another thing,

Marsha was my very best friend. How could anything be wrong between best friends?

So I let her hands stray over my breasts. I was even tempted to touch her the same way, but I was too awkward to try it. A little while later, we stopped kissing and she took her hands away. "I'm sorry, Frances," she said. "I just couldn't help myself." I felt myself blushing a little as I murmured that it was okay.

After that, we ended up kissing and caressing almost every time we got together. I realized that it had gone beyond the bounds of friendship, but the word "lesbian" never really entered my mind until one day Marsha used it. She explained that she had always known she was different from the other girls. She had no sexual interest at all in boys, but only in other women. I was a little shocked by her admission. The word she used to describe herself was one that, previously, I had only heard used with contempt, or as part of a dirty joke.

I was very confused, because even though I did like boys and found myself sexually attracted to them, I also enjoyed Marsha's touch. By now, I also enjoyed touching her. Did that mean that I was a lesbian, too? While I was struggling with that thought, Marsha said, "You know, Frances, you're obviously straight. Women like me know about those things. I can tell the difference between a straight woman and a lesbian a mile away. But that doesn't mean we can't enjoy each other's company and even sexual contact with each other."

I was too embarrassed by the subject to continue, and Marsha sensed this. Immediately, she took me in her arms and kissed me. I allowed myself to melt into her caress. A few months later, while I was visiting her, we found ourselves naked and in bed together. She kissed my body all over and brought me to my very first orgasm with her fingers, lips, and tongue. I didn't know such pleasure was possible.

Not long after that, I started seeing a young man rather seriously and ended up having sex with him. It was good, but not as tender or loving as what I had experienced in Marsha's arms. I continued seeing him, and we even talked about marriage. I also visited Marsha regularly and had sex with her as well.

After I broke up with him, which didn't take very long, I saw more and more of Marsha. Our lovemaking got very intense at times, and I often wondered if I wasn't really a lesbian, too. Every time I asked Marsha about that, though, she assured me that I was not. Sometimes, it was obvious that she wished I were.

I didn't see much of Marsha after I left for college. Every time I went home I'd manage to visit with her. We'd always end up in bed. While I was away, I had relationships with several men, and had sex with most of them. None of them lived up to what I had come to expect from Marsha.

Then I met Albert. He was a few years older than I and majoring in science, while I was studying liberal arts. He was a little shy. We had one humanities class together. I knew from the way he looked at me that he was interested. I was aware for quite a while that he wanted to ask me out. Finally, after class one day, he got up the nerve. Rather awkwardly, he asked if I'd care to have a pizza with him that evening. I said I would.

We had a good time. Once the initial awkwardness had passed, Albert turned out to be a very interesting person. After a few dates, we ended up making love. It was good. Very good. His sexual skills made up for his social backwardness. He made me feel absolutely wonderful, bringing me to orgasm after orgasm. It was so good, that I didn't think once about Marsha.

After that, we got closer and closer. About a year later, we decided to get married. I wasn't sure how I'd break the news to Marsha, but I knew I had to do it. So I made a special trip home, just to see her. When I went to her place, her face lit up. She took me in her arms and kissed me passionately. I gently broke the embrace. "Marsha," I began. "I have to tell you something."

"Let me guess," she said with a titter. "You've decided to marry Albert."

"Why, yes," I answered. "How did you know?"

"It's been obvious," she answered. "From our phone conversations and your very infrequent letters. I'm very happy for you. Congratulations."

At first I didn't know whether she really meant it. But one look in her eyes convinced me. Then she took me in her arms again and kissed me. Before I knew it, we were in bed together, making love like we always did. It was fabulous.

After I dressed and as I was leaving, I noticed a painting on her wall of a nude woman that I had never seen before. I recognized Marsha's style. I stared at it for a moment without saying a word. "I recently found somebody, too," Marsha said softly. "Her name is Virginia. She's a doctor. We are very much in love." She looked at me as though waiting for my approval.

"That's great," I said, really meaning it. "Now we can all be happy."

"Yes," Marsha said, wistfully. "As long as you and I can keep what we have."

In spite of what she said, I made a conscious effort to stay away from her for the first year or so of my marriage. I knew that if I saw her we would end up having sex. I didn't want to start my marriage off by having an affair, even if it was with another woman. After a while, though, I found myself missing her desperately. Missing the loving that she gave me. That special loving that I only got from her.

I told Albert that I was going to visit my mother for a few days and went back to my hometown. I knew that he couldn't get away from his job, so I would be on my own. As soon as I got home, I called Marsha, and she invited me over. When I knocked at her door, I was surprised to have it opened by a woman I didn't know.

She smiled brightly and said, "Hi, I'm Virginia. Marsha has told me so much about you. Please come in." At first I wondered if Marsha had told her everything. I was soon comforted to understand that she had not. We spent a pleasant hour or so chatting, until Virginia said that she had to leave. She was on duty at the hospital that night. Minutes after she was out the door, Marsha and I were embracing and heading for the bedroom. Our sex was fantastic, as usual. I made love with her three more times before I had to return to my everyday life.

After that, Marsha and I saw each other whenever we could. Sometimes months would go by between get-togethers, but we always remained close, at least on the phone. Then, about a year ago, she and Virginia moved to this city. That makes it a lot easier for us to meet. We've been doing so about once every week or two. I just got back from her place now.

I have nothing negative to say about Albert. He's a great husband and still a great lover. But Marsha and I share something very special. So special that there's no one else who could ever satisfy the need that she fills for me. I love Albert in one way and I love Marsha in another.

I wish this were the kind of world in which people—especially Albert—could understand the difference between the love that can exist between a woman and a man and the love that can exist between two women. I dream about telling Albert and getting his approval for my love of Marsha, but I know that isn't realistic. In the meantime, I'm living in two perfect worlds. I guess as long as my relationship with Marsha remains a secret, I'll continue to do so.

ELEVEN
Discovered

No matter how intent people are on keeping their secret desires unspoken, it is inevitable that some will be caught. Eventually, the most carefully guarded and cautiously undisclosed sexual practices and fantasies may be discovered by a life-partner. This chapter tells the stories of two people who had the experience of being caught.

As you might expect, one of them was devastated by the discovery. In fact, it spelled the end of her marriage. Olga tried to keep her obsession with Internet exhibitionism from her husband, but that turned out to be impossible. Now she regrets having been so careless in indulging her private desire.

On the other hand, Craig says getting caught was the best thing that ever happened to him. For years, he hid his desire to surreptitiously observe others as they engaged in sexual activity. He could not hide it forever, though. When his wife found him out, the result was somewhat surprising.

Webcam

Olga had just turned forty when she told us about herself. She is five feet nine inches tall, with long, straight, blond hair that comes almost to her waist, and round blue-gray eyes. Although her figure is not outstanding, when she speaks she has a way of throwing her shoulders back that seems designed to call attention to her breasts. Unfettered by an undergarment, they stand out proudly against the front of her sweater, her nipples erect and clearly outlined. She talks unhesitatingly about her personal life, including its disappointments.

I really love Morley, but it's hopeless now. He wants a divorce. Nothing I can say will change his mind. In a way, I can't say I blame him. He's somewhat older than I am and was set in his ways even when I first met him. We've been married for five years. He knew then that I had a lot of sexual experience and that I was interested in some things that he regarded as kinky. He accepted all that. Now he feels that I have betrayed him. I guess that's what made him decide to end our marriage.

The trouble started about a year ago, when I got a home computer. At first, I didn't know what I was going to do with the thing. Everybody else has one, so I thought I needed one, too. I tried using it to do our taxes, but that turned out to be a nightmare. Then I thought maybe I would write a book. I don't work and I don't have a lot of friends, so I had plenty of time on my hands. I soon discovered, though, that I had nothing to write about.

Then I started learning about the Internet. It really is amazing. It's a giant network that somehow puts all the computers in the world in touch with each other. There's lots of information available on the Internet, but I found I was most interested in interaction with other people.

First I found the chat rooms. These are Internet locations where groups of people can have typewritten conversations with each other instantaneously. I especially liked the idea that it was so anonymous. Everybody used an Internet ID or nickname, and usually that's all you got to know about anybody you were conversing with. Most of the time, the chat ended up centering about sex. People made all kinds of obscene proposals to each other, knowing that they'd never really meet or even know who they were talking to.

Then I learned about CU-SeeMe reflectors. These are like chat rooms, except they are for people with special little cameras. They can actually see each other as they chat. I gathered that the sex in these reflectors was even more explicit than in the chat rooms, so I went right out and bought one of the cameras. It cost less than a hundred dollars.

When I got it plugged in and up and running, I connected with one of the reflectors. Within minutes, I was hooked, like an addict. I saw men and women and couples all doing sexy things and typing messages to each other about it. Some would be taking their clothes off, exhibiting themselves to strangers by computer. Others would actually be having sex. Lots of the time cameras would be focused on women giving oral sex to their male partners. That really turned me on.

I guess the biggest turn-on came when I decided to stop just "lurking" (which means watching) and to participate, myself. I had always liked wearing sexy clothes and showing off, but hadn't done much of that since my marriage to Morley. Now, I felt free to show off in an even more explicit way. Pointing my camera at the front of my blouse, I began unbuttoning it. I started receiving typewritten messages from other people in the group encouraging me.

"Show those titties," one of them wrote.

"Yes, SxyScan (that was my Internet nickname, for sexy Scandinavian), keep going."

The words of these strangers really excited me, so I did keep going. As you can see, I don't usually wear a bra. When my blouse was open, my breasts were visible to all the others in the reflector. It gave me thrills I couldn't describe. Unconsciously, I reached down and began stroking myself, masturbating right through my clothes. I was glad that particular part of me was out of camera range, because at that point I would have been embarrassed to do that in front of strangers. I did remove my blouse completely, though. After a while, I even played a little with my nipples where everybody could see me.

That night, when Morley came home, I was so turned on that I practically raped him. We made ferocious love, tearing the sheets right off the bed. The whole time, I kept thinking about what I had experienced on the Internet that day. When we finished making love, I still wasn't satisfied. After Morley fell asleep, I masturbated until I was completely worn out.

The next day, as soon as Morley left for work, I was in front of the computer, going back to the sexy chat room. I didn't even bother to get dressed. I just sat there in my nightgown, looking forward to exposing myself the way I had done the day before. I was disappointed to find that the reflector was empty. Nobody there but me.

So I started surfing around until I found more reflectors. Soon I was showing my breasts to strangers again. This time, I repositioned the camera and showed my pubic area as well. I really enjoyed the comments I received from the people who were watching. Even more than that, I enjoyed the feeling it gave me to show myself to strangers. Once again that night, Morley and I had very hot sex. I think my secret exhibitionism turned me on more than the actual sex with Morley did.

About a week later, I discovered Webcams. A Webcam is a camera that some man or woman places in his or her bedroom and is hooked up to the Internet. The camera takes a picture every thirty seconds or every two minutes, or whatever it's set for, and broadcasts it over the Internet to anyone who cares to watch it. I found one that a woman had set up in her bathroom, so the whole world could watch her taking a shower or even peeing whenever she was in there. There was another one set up in someone's living room. During the day, you could observe them doing ordinary family activities, like watching TV with their kids and stuff like that. In the evenings, after their kids were in bed, you'd usually see them making out, or even having sex, on the living room couch.

Peeking into the lives of the people who had Webcams was very exciting. Pretty soon, I found myself thinking about what it would be like to have a Webcam of my own. I found out that there are companies that will set one up for you and even publicize it. They charge a fee to people who want to watch, controlling it by issuing secret passwords that are needed to make the connection. I contacted one of them and said that I wanted to set up a Webcam. In return, they promised me a percentage of what they collected. I was really doing this for the thrill of exhibitionism, but the idea of monetary compensation added to the excitement, because it meant there were people who would be paying to look at me. That made it even more thrilling.

My Webcam was up and running in just a few days. It was different from the reflectors, because this was strictly one-way. I could not see the people who were watching me and I had no idea of how many of them there were. I never even knew, at any particular time, whether there was anybody watching at all. I could shut off the cam if I ever wanted some privacy, but when it was on, I had no way of knowing whether I had an audience. I just assumed that I always did.

I liked having the camera on me at all times. In the beginning, I would sit in front of the cam and deliberately expose myself in as provocative a way as I could. After a while, I just accepted the Webcam as a silent eye on my life. I did a lot more dressing and undressing than I used to, and I spent a lot more time walking around in the nude. Also, I masturbated a lot more, usually while lying naked on my bed. It really heated me up to know that there were people out there watching as I did so. But I stopped playing directly for the audience. I always shut the cam down before Morley got home.

Morley is very conservative about the privacy of sex. He always got angry if I wore clothing that he thought was too revealing. Even cleavage or a short skirt would set him off on a jealous rampage. I knew that if he found out about the Webcam, he would have a fit. I wasn't too worried, though, because I knew he was not interested in computers. In fact, he was downright anti-computer and wouldn't have anything to do with them.

I realized that exhibitionism was important to me; that it filled every minute of my life with sexual excitement. I knew that if I exhibited myself in person to anyone at all, Morley would go through the roof. But I figured that he would never find out about my computer activities, as long as I kept my kinky desires to myself and my Webcam audience.

After a while, I started leaving the cam on at night, when Morley and I were making love. My activities during the day made me hungry for sex. So, most nights, as soon as he got home we would get right down to it. I must admit that when we were actually making love, the knowledge that there were strangers watching on their computer screens brought me to new heights of sexual arousal. Sometimes, I would do things to Morley that made him very glad. I was really performing for my unseen audience.

I liked taking his penis halfway into my mouth and turning to face the camera, so that the people watching would get a nice detailed view of the head I was giving him. Sometimes, when I sensed that he was about to have an orgasm, I would remove him from my mouth so the camera could capture the spurts as they shot through the air. If I could, I'd move so they would splash across my breasts. Then I'd turn and spread my legs, so the viewers could get a good, close-up view of my genitals. It kept me sizzling hot, and Morley never suspected a thing.

When I received my first check from the company that had set me up, it was more than I expected it to be. It sort of validated what I was doing, giving me the feeling that my hidden need for exhibitionism was okay, even valuable. If it kept up, I'd have my computer paid for in three months. Best of all, it meant there were lots of people out there paying to look at me naked and paying to watch me and my husband having sex. I felt like a movie star, a cyber-celebrity.

Of course, that turned out to be the problem. I realized that my performances could be seen on computers all over the country; all over the world, even. I forgot that they could also be seen on computers in my own neighborhood.

One day, one of Morley's friends at work said something to him about seeing his act on the Webcam the night before. Morley didn't know what he was talking about and said so. Pretty soon, his friend had given him an Internet education, and Morley knew everything. His friend even tuned in during the afternoon to actually show him what I was doing when he wasn't home. I can only imagine how shocked my husband was to see me stretching out naked on our bed and stroking myself in front of the Webcam.

That same afternoon, he came home in a frenzy and shouted, "Where is it?" I didn't know what he was talking about until he started kicking my computer, smashing it to pieces. "The camera," he yelled. "Where is it?"

I was speechless. He started looking around the room frantically, pulling things off shelves and tearing the drapes, searching for the cam. Finally, in silence, I pointed to it and watched as he threw it onto the floor and ground it to a pulp with his heel. Then, without a word, he tossed a few things in a suitcase and walked out of the house.

That was two months ago. He still hasn't returned. We've had a couple of conversations on the phone, but all we talk about is the property settlement. Last week, he had me served with divorce papers.

I feel terrible about the way our marriage ended. Sometimes, I ask myself whether things would have been better if I had told my husband about my hidden desire as soon as I discovered it. I fantasize about the two of us surfing the Internet together, deliberately putting on sexual exhibitions for strangers on reflectors, or even on the Webcam. If only he could have understood, like so many of the men I've seen on the screen, we could have had a wonderful and completely satisfying marriage.

I realize, of course, that never could have been. There are some things a person should never let her husband find out about her. What I needed was something he never could have given me. Maybe I could have gotten it anyway. If only I had been more careful.

Telescopes

*C*raig, twenty-six, works in a travel agency, although he says he has not yet done any traveling. His sandy-colored hair and blue eyes give him a Dennis the Menace look, and a kind of boyish charm. He speaks frankly, but there are times when the things he is saying embarrass him, and his face reddens.

I've kept my little hangup a secret all my life, but I should have known that one day I'd get caught. As it happens, getting caught was one of the best things that ever happened to me. The way I see it, getting caught was probably what got the whole thing started.

I was a little kid. When my parents went out for the evening, I had a baby-sitter named Riane. She was about in her late teens. I kind of liked her. She seemed to understand me, even though she seemed a million years old at the time.

One night, when I was supposed to be asleep, I thought I heard her talking to someone in the living room. I crept out of my room, curious to see what I was missing. When I got halfway down the stairs, I was able to see the living room couch. Riane was sitting there with a boyfriend. They were giggling and kidding around, but what caught my attention more than anything was that her blouse was open. I still remember the feeling I got when I saw her crisp white bra and her big, firm breasts overflowing it. My mother was very modest and always careful to close her door when she was dressing, so this was the first time I had seen that much female anatomy. I was fascinated.

I just stood there staring as the boyfriend removed the bra completely to begin kissing and sucking on Riane's nipples. I couldn't take my eyes off the scene. I thought I saw Riane's hand going for the front of his pants. I was wondering what that was all about, when suddenly she looked up and spotted me.

"Oh!" she shrieked. "You little sneak. Get down here this instant." By the time I got to the living room, she was totally dressed again. "You've been very nasty," she scolded. "What do you think would happen if your mother found out about this?"

Actually, I had no idea. It had never occurred to me that what I had been doing was wrong. I was just learning about the world around me by keeping my eyes and ears open. But Riane made me feel that there was something especially naughty about watching them on the couch. Seeing her with her blouse open and seeing her boyfriend touching her that way wasn't the same as seeing other things. It was "nasty." It made me a "sneak."

I begged her not to tell my mother. After giving me a thorough scolding, she promised that she wouldn't. I went back to bed whimpering in shame. But as soon as I had settled down in the dark, I found myself thinking about what I had seen. It certainly inflamed my curiosity. Somehow, knowing how wrong it was made it seem all the more fascinating.

I was too scared to try peeking at them again that night, but I decided that I would do so the next time she baby-sat me. It was maybe a week later. This time, I deliberately stayed awake after she put me to bed. I listened as she sat on the couch watching television. Eventually, I heard a soft knock at the front door and someone else coming in. After waiting a while, I stole quietly down the stairs to have a look.

It was the boyfriend again. He and Riane were kissing, and his hands were roaming all over her. Without quite understanding why, I was hoping that he would take off her blouse and bra again, but that didn't happen. I just stood there for a long time watching them kiss, and then crept back to my room.

For some reason, I couldn't get to sleep after that. I was still fascinated by what I had seen, but more importantly, I was excited by the idea that I had done something "nasty" and got away with it. I think the seeds of my voyeurism were planted that night.

In my teens, I found myself driven by the need to observe other people when they didn't know they were being watched. I remember borrowing some tools from the wood shop at my high school and drilling a hole through an unused fire-exit door in the girls' locker room. When I wasn't there to look through it, I plugged it with a piece of wood that I cut specially for the purpose. When I was there, I removed the wood and watched as the girls dressed, and undressed, and showered, and dried themselves off, before and after their gym classes. I never told anyone about my peephole; not even my closest friends. I just knew that they would disapprove of anything so "sneaky" and "nasty."

Sometimes, I would play hooky from my classes so I could squint through the little hole at the girls I went to school with. It thrilled me to see their budding pink nipples and the sparse hair that was sprouting between their legs. I liked it when they bent over with their asses facing me and I could see everything all at once.

I didn't have a girlfriend. I didn't even go out with girls. But as the other guys talked about their exploits, I wasn't the least bit jealous or envious. I had my secret peephole, and it was all I needed to keep me sexually satisfied.

Most of the time, I would see my fill, and then go off to the boys' bathroom and lock myself in a stall to whack off, my head reeling with the images I had just seen. Occasionally, when I was sure I wouldn't be caught, I would take out my dick while watching and jack off right there on the spot. That was the most exciting of all—peeping as a turn-on—with instant gratification in the form of masturbation.

When I got older, I started dating. I had sex with a few girls and always found it satisfying, but not as satisfying as peeping. Sometimes, after dropping off my date, I would go cruising the neighborhood in my car, hoping for a nasty glimpse through someone's bedroom window. Once in a while, I'd take a girl to a local lovers' lane. We'd neck in the car, but I was always more interested in trying to get a look at what was going on in the cars around us. I was very careful, though, knowing that if the girl I was with caught me at it, she'd think I was a perverted sneak and be filled with contempt for my nasty ways.

I didn't have any special feelings for any of the girls I went out with until I met Kay. I don't exactly know what it was, but there was something between us right from the start. We had good times together. After we had been dating for only a few weeks we started having great sex. I didn't tell her about my perversion, because I didn't want to screw up what was starting to look like a wonderful relationship.

I still looked for every possible opportunity to peep into other people's sex lives. After Kay and I were married, I even tried to bring that sizzling voyeuristic excitement into our home life. When she was in the shower, I'd open the bathroom door just a crack and position myself outside the room so I could see her reflection in the bathroom mirror. It made me nervous, because I was always afraid she would catch me at it and think I was a nasty little pervert. Besides, I don't know how I would have explained that I found it more exciting to sneak a look at her that way than to walk right into the room and watch her openly. So I usually only did it for a few minutes at a time.

Shortly after we were married, we moved to our present apartment. Kay was in love with the kitchen, but I picked

it for the view. Our living room windows face a tall resi-
dential complex, with lots and lots of windows to look
into. I just knew there would be lots of opportunities for
me to window shop. I even bought a pair of high-powered
binoculars.

For the first few months, I used my binoculars only when
Kay was out for some reason. I used to get the shakes from
some of the things I saw. There were two women in an apartment across the way who used to exercise in the nude every
evening after work. I would focus my binoculars on them
and watch their tits bouncing up and down as they worked
out to some video they put on the TV. There were a couple
of gay men who seemed totally unaware that they could be
seen while giving each other blowjobs. There was a college
girl who enjoyed having two or three men come in and fuck
her on the same night.

After a while, I found that just watching when Kay was
out didn't satisfy me. So I'd start getting up in the middle
of the night and slip out of bed to take up my position in
front of the living room window. Then, binoculars at the
ready, I'd scan the building across the street, my expert eye
searching for telltale signs that this window or that one
would yield rewards. I got to see the intimate details of
more people's lives than you can imagine. Never a dull
moment.

It got to be kind of a ritual. I'd make a few sounds like
I was coming out of a deep sleep and wait to see if there
was any response from Kay. Then I'd get up and head for
the kitchen for a drink of water. If she hadn't called out
to me by that time, I'd figure I was safe and spend an
hour or so peeking into windows. Kay is a heavy sleeper.
Most of the time, she never even knew I had gotten out
of bed.

I remember one close call, though. I was sitting in an
easy chair in the unlit living room, staring through my binoculars at a woman in her fifties or so who was lying on
her bed, playing with herself. My own cock was hard as a

197

rock, and I was rubbing it up and down. I was wishing I could go in and wake my wife up for some sizzling sex, but I was afraid to because I thought she might wonder what had heated me up so much. I was paranoid enough to think she might even figure it out. So I just sat there staring and beating off, when, suddenly I heard a sound from the bedroom. Kay was getting out of bed, calling, "Craig? Craig, where are you?"

I got my cock back into my shorts with the speed of lightning, and none to soon. Before I knew it, she was standing next to me with the light on. "What are you doing in here?" she asked, rubbing her eyes. "Having trouble sleeping?"

I took the easy out she had handed me. "Yeah," I murmured, hiding the binoculars under the chair cushion. "I was tossing and turning, so I decided to sit up for a while."

"Well, come on back to bed," she said. "I'll help you fall asleep." As soon as we got back into bed, she started giving me a blowjob. I was so excited from what I had been watching that I got off within a few seconds. After that, I fell right to sleep.

For a couple of weeks after that, I resisted the urge to get up at night for another peeping session. But something inside was clawing at me. Life just didn't seem complete unless I could indulge my secret passion. Eventually, I gave in to it again, standing night after night in front of the living room window as my wife snored softly inside. Some nights, I saw nothing at all, but there was still a special kind of thrill in trying. Just knowing that I might get lucky was enough to keep me inflamed.

Then, one night about three months ago, the unthinkable happened. I had gotten quietly out of bed and was standing by the window. In the building across the street, a man and woman were having some kind of argument, throwing things at each other and waving their arms wildly in the air. I had never seen either of them before. Until now, their shades were always closed. Suddenly, in the middle of their fight, they started tearing each other's clothes off. At first, I thought I was going to see a murder, but instead they started making furiously passionate sex.

The sight of it was so exciting that my cock sprang to full erection and worked its way out of the fly in my boxer shorts. One hand held the binoculars pressed to my eyes, but the other began stroking my hard-on. I think I was making the strokes coincide with the movements of the man in the window, who was entering the woman from behind and moving his hips rhythmically in and out.

I was so engrossed in what I was seeing and doing that I was totally unaware that Kay had gotten out of bed and come into the living room to investigate. She flipped on the light for a second and then shut it off. I knew she had seen everything. I was caught. If she stayed with me at all, my marriage would never be the same.

I turned to face her, my mind racing as I tried to think of some innocent explanation. But she didn't give me a chance. Instead, she reached out and put her hand on my cock. "Oh, I don't ever remember it being so big," she said. "What have you been watching?"

Embarrassed, but not knowing what else to do, I began telling her about the neighbors, and their fight, and how it had turned into sex. I could tell by the way she was breathing that the description was exciting her. "Here," I said, handing her the binoculars. "See for yourself."

She took the binoculars and focused them on the window that I pointed out to her. For a long time, she just stood there staring, breathing hard, but not saying a word. Then, slowly, she handed the glasses back to me. "Here," she said. "You can clearly see the woman's pussy now. I want you to look and tell me everything you see."

I couldn't believe this was really happening. Flabbergasted, I turned back to the window to follow her instructions. As I raised the binoculars to my eyes, I felt Kay's fingers wrapping around the shaft of my hard, but getting harder, dick. I began to describe the dark bush of hair that surrounded the other woman's pussy. I talked in detail about her nipples, how hard and swollen they looked. I spoke about the size of the man's cock and the way it looked as he slipped it between the cheeks of the woman's ass.

The more I talked, the harder Kay stroked me. I felt an orgasm rising and wasn't sure how she would feel about me coming this way. I struggled against it, but she seemed determined to bring it on. She kept jerking and pulling at my cock until I had no choice. Then, just as it was about to spit, she dropped to her knees and positioned her mouth so that I would come right into it.

The cum seemed to go on forever. It was the best I ever had in my whole life up till then. When it was done, I was so grateful that I ate her out right there on the living room rug until she came again and again.

By the time we dragged ourselves back to bed, we were so fatigued that we fell asleep without another word. The next morning, when I left for work, Kay was still sleeping. When I came home that night, she had a surprise for me. Set up in front of the living room window were two wide-range telescopes. When I saw them, I stared in disbelief. She just giggled and said, "His and hers."

Since then, we have spent lots of nights together, looking at the urban landscape through our telescopes and hoping to find some good action. If she spots something I haven't seen, she tells me about it, so I can focus my scope on the same window. I do the same for her. It seems that both of us are turned on by the same thing. Sometimes we get so excited by our peeping that we fuck and suck each other until we're practically unconscious. It keeps getting better all the time.

That's why I say getting caught turned out to be the best thing that ever happened to me. If it wasn't for that, I probably would have kept this nasty desire of mine a secret forever. I would have lived in constant fear that my wife would find out, Eventually, that would have driven a wedge between us. Now it's more like a hobby that we both share. It heats up our love life like nothing else ever could.

TWELVE
I Found a Partner

*M*ost of the people whose stories are told in this book nurture secret desires that remain unspoken. Many believe that if they were to divulge their hidden fantasies to their mates, disaster would result. As we saw from the experience of Olga in the previous chapter, that is sometimes true. The result, however, is that, for too many persons, life becomes a kind of torment, a battle between the way things are and the way they would like things to be.

It sometimes happens, though, that there is a perfect partner out there, just waiting to be discovered, another person who harbors the same secret desire and is looking for a mate with whom to share it. An old expression says, "There's someone for everyone." This is as true of sexual proclivities as it is of appearance, intellect, or any other human trait.

The people in this chapter found their partners. For Heather, it was a co-worker who had the same interest as she and with whom she can indulge her secret desire while remaining true to her husband. For Preston, it was a woman who wanted the same things he did, although for different reasons. Together, they found love and perfect satisfaction.

Not everyone will be successful in finding a match for their own peculiarities. We offer the stories in this chapter as examples of the happiness people can attain when they do succeed in doing so. Perhaps the experiences described by Heather and Preston can furnish a goal toward which readers may strive.

Manual Labors

*A*t thirty-three, Heather is rather well-known among lawyers in her area. She is a deputy public defender, employed by the taxpayers to represent persons accused of crime who are unable to afford their own attorneys. She is quite attractive, with long, straight, sandy blond hair and hazel eyes framed by fashionable designer glasses. She is tall, with a thin but curvaceous figure. Walking among the holding cells located in the basement of the criminal court building, she is usually greeted by a chorus of whistles and catcalls. When the prisoners learn that she is there to defend one of them, however, they become quietly respectful.

I'll admit I like the excitement of dealing with criminal types and low-class individuals. It's fun when they act like a bunch of horny animals at the first sight of me and then settle down as soon as they realize who and what I am. Their very freedom depends on my abilities, and they know it.

My husband, Gary, is a more respectable type. He's got a flourishing and lucrative personal-injury practice. Gary's idea of living dangerously is to hold out for a higher offer from some insurance company adjuster. We get along fine. They say opposites attract. Gary and I have a satisfying sex life, but, frankly, I still masturbate quite a lot.

I've always loved masturbating. I can't even remember when I first started. It's just something I've always done. I like knowing that I have the power to give myself the incredible feeling of orgasm, whenever and wherever I want. Sometimes, at the courthouse, I go into the ladies' room and masturbate in one of the stalls. Once, I even did it there during a ten-minute comfort break while I was on trial.

When I was a teenager, my best friend, Rhonda, and I used to masturbate together. It started one night when she was sleeping over at my house. We were in separate beds, of course, and the lights were out. I thought she was asleep, so I went ahead and diddled myself, like I usually did when going to bed. At some point, I thought I heard a familiar sound coming from Rhonda's bed. I stopped what I was doing and held my breath to listen. I heard the unmistakable sound of fingers moving in a wet vagina and I knew my friend was doing the same thing as I.

I didn't say anything about it until the following morning, when I told her what I had heard. She laughed and said that she had heard me doing it and that's what got her started. The next time we spent the night together, we left the light on and watched each other. Watching her do it and at the same time knowing that she was watching me do it made it all the more exciting.

After that, we masturbated together regularly, every chance we got. But adolescent girls grow up, and before long, we were going out with boys. Somehow, it didn't seem right after that, and we did it less and less. Eventually, Rhonda got a steady boyfriend and started spending all her time with him. I had boyfriends, too. So my masturbation went back to being a solitary pursuit.

Even when I became sexually active with the boys and young men I was dating, I continued masturbating. When I was in college and law school, there would be times I'd have sex with some guy I was seeing and then go right back to my room to masturbate. On a few occasions, I tried doing it while making love with a partner. As he thrust in and out of me, I'd rub my clit with the tip of my middle finger. I could sense that it made them resentful, though.

Most of the men didn't mention it, but one did. He said,

"Hey, what's the matter, isn't my cock good enough for you?" I tried to explain that touching myself improved the experience for me, but he became offended. Before long, I got the point, and restricted my auto-eroticism to the privacy of my own room.

By the time I met Gary, I had learned to keep that little secret to myself. We started dating when I was in my last year of law school and Gary was a first-year associate with one of the large personal-injury firms. We fell in love and decided to get married as soon as I finished school. Our love life was excellent. Gary is a better lover than any man I've ever known.

Soon after we got married, I decided to see how he'd feel about my masturbation. One night, while we were making love, I reached down and started fingering myself. We were kissing at the time, and his hands were caressing my breasts. I was wearing a very flimsy nightgown and he was nude. At first, I just quietly rubbed my slit, carrying a little of the moisture up to my clit. Then, to make sure he'd notice, I moaned a little. Taking his hand, I put it right over mine, so he could feel me doing things to myself.

He gently pulled my hand away and replaced it with his own, stroking and petting my vagina lovingly. I thought he had misunderstood me, that maybe when I put his hand on top of mine, he thought I was asking him to take over. So I slid my hand under his and started stroking myself again. This time, I slipped one finger deep into my vulva, rotating it in time to the groans that were issuing from my throat.

I really wanted him to understand how exciting it was for me to masturbate with him right there to watch me and to do other things to me while I played with myself. But he just didn't seem to get the point. Once again, he removed my hand and replaced it with his own, driving his finger inside me and moving it in and out like a miniature penis. It felt good. I just placed my hand over his and started rubbing my clit while he screwed me with his finger.

This time, he became angry. "Look," he said. "I can figure

out what to do. You don't have to show me every step of the way. I know how to please you, don't I?"

"Of course," I murmured softly. "But I like touching myself, too."

He acted as if he didn't hear me. "All right, then," he said, with an air of finality. "Let me do things my way." He went back to stroking and petting me, but the mood was broken. Taking hold of his penis, I guided it into me and lay back to let him finish. Later as he slept beside me, I lay awake for hours, feeling frustrated, but afraid that if I masturbated he would wake up and be angry. That night I realized that masturbation would never be part of my marital sex-play. I must admit I was disappointed.

Maybe that's why I developed a kind of attitude about it. Like a crusader. It came out one evening, after I offered a ride home to Ruth, one of the secretaries who works in the office. When we got to her house, she told me her husband was out with their son and invited me in for a cold drink. I accepted, sensing there was something on her mind. As we sat on her living room couch sipping lemonade, she said, "I'd like to ask your advice about a little problem I have."

"Sure," I said, thinking it was probably a legal matter.

"Well," she began, "I'm pretty sure my son has started masturbating, and I don't quite know what to do about it. My husband is very much against it, and I'm afraid to tell him, because I know he'd fly off the handle and traumatize the boy. But I don't want him to develop bad habits. What do you think?"

Suddenly, I saw a soapbox before me. "I'll tell you what I think," I said as if I were summing up to a jury. "I don't think there's anything wrong with masturbation. The problem isn't masturbation, it's society's repressive attitude about masturbation. God damn it, it's good, clean, healthy fun. Why should you stop him? I do it myself, every chance I get." I felt my face turning red and realized I had said more than I should have.

For a moment, there was utter silence in the room. Then,

in a soft voice, Ruth said, "You do? I thought you were married."

I felt defensive. "What does one thing have to do with the other?" I asked rhetorically. "You're married. Now tell the truth, don't you ever feel like masturbating?"

"I did it a lot when I was younger," she said. "But I always thought you were supposed to give that up when you became an adult." There was something about the way she said it and about the rosy color that seemed to be staining her ears that made me think she wasn't being entirely candid.

"I don't know why that should be," I said. "Adults have just as much sex drive as adolescents. Why should we deprive ourselves of our innocent pleasures? I like doing it, and I don't mind saying so." As I spoke, I realized that until that moment, I never had said so. Not to anybody.

Ruth took a deep breath. "When you do it," she began. "How do you do it?"

"Well," I stammered. "I . . . er, I . . . er, usually it's when I . . ." I didn't really know what to say.

"Would you show me?" she asked. Her voice was so soft that I wasn't sure I had heard her. I just stared. She cleared her throat and said it again, this time slightly louder. "Would you show me?"

If I had stopped to think things over, I never would have done what I did next. I would have taken the conservative route, changed the subject, and gotten out of there to go back to my safe little world. But her words brought back memories of my adolescent experiences. Deep memories. The kind they call cell memories. I was flooded with that feeling of excitement that I used to get whenever I prepared to masturbate with Rhonda.

Without letting thought get in the way, I leaned way back against the cushions of the couch and worked my skirt up over my hips. I felt Ruth's eyes on me, watching in silence as I slid my pantyhose down and kicked them off with my feet. All that covered me now was the dampening crotch of a pair of pale pink panties.

I started rubbing myself through the material, feeling just a little strange about exposing my vagina to Ruth. But it felt so good to be stroking myself in front of her that, a moment later, I pulled the wet crotch to one side and began diddling myself in earnest. I drove first one and then two fingers deep inside me, rotating them and moaning slightly at the pleasure that it brought. It made me want to reveal myself completely to her view. With a swift movement of my hands, I pulled the panties off and spread my legs wide, showing her my open vulva.

I was so wet I could feel moisture oozing from inside me to coat my thighs, as I plunged my fingers back into my slit. My clit was swollen and hard. Every movement of my hand brought one of my knuckles against it. As I masturbated, I looked directly into Ruth's eyes. The sight of her watching made the whole experience even more exciting.

Without taking her gaze from my frothy vulva, Ruth stood up and fumbled with the front of her pants. When she had them unbuttoned, she hooked her thumbs into the waistband and pulled pants and panties down with a single motion, exposing a thick, dark bush of curling hair. "Yes," she murmured. "Keep doing it." With that, she sat back down on the couch, spread her own legs, and began stroking herself.

Her vagina looked like a huge red gash, with thick lips surrounding it and tendrils of coarse hair growing all around it. The clitoral hood moved back on its own accord, revealing the swollen purple knob of her clit. With a strangled gasp, she started rolling it, pushing it gently back and forth between her index and middle finger. Seeing her perform this intimate act and knowing that she was seeing me at the same time raised me to a height of arousal that I had not known since my adolescent years.

"Oh, Ruth," I whispered. "Let me see you put your finger in it." She complied at once, inserting her middle finger deep into her opening and thrusting it in and out. Each time it came forth, I could see the coating of shining juices that it had picked up from her vulva. Each time it went in, I could see the lips of her vagina clinging to it, caressing it.

"Now your clit," I said. "Touch your clit again." She continued frigging herself with her finger, but immediately brought her other hand into play, using it to tease and pet her eager button. Having her respond to my suggestions made me feel even hotter. I longed to have her give me direction, too.

As if she read my mind, she said, "Open yourself for me. Let me look inside." Her words were like an instant aphrodisiac. I used my fingers to pull the lips of my vulva apart as she had instructed, feeling a rush of fluid coating all my membranes and flowing out onto my hands. I knew my orgasm was building. The thought of having her watch me come was tantalizingly erotic. I wanted to be sure she knew.

"Oh, I'm going to come," I murmured. "I'm going to come while you watch."

"Yes," she encouraged. "Come for me. And watch me. I'll come for you at the same time." With that, her body started to thrash, her bare bottom flailing against the couch and her hips moving in jerky little circles. Her fingers drove deeper and more rhythmically into her sex, and she started to chant, "I'm coming. I'm coming. I'm coming. I'm coming."

It was all too much for me. I too began to climax. Wanting to excite her the way she was exciting me, I announced it as well. "Oh, yeah. Oh, yeah. I'm coming with you. I'm coming too. I'm going to explode."

We continued rubbing ourselves and making deep guttural sounds for what seemed like an hour, but was probably less than a minute. Then at last, we both started to calm down. I was afraid that one or both of us would feel some kind of remorse afterwards, but I was wrong. As Ruth stood up and dressed, she said, "That was wonderful. I haven't had an experience like that since I was a teenager."

I laughed. "Neither have I," I said, trying to rearrange my own clothing. It turned out that, like me, Ruth had a girlfriend with whom she masturbated as an adolescent. We learned that we had a great deal in common. Like me, she longed for the innocent excitement of those days of mutual watching. She also had attempted to interest her husband in playing that kind of game. But he was totally opposed to masturbation, even more than Gary. So she had stifled her desires and kept them to herself. Suddenly, we had each found a kindred spirit, a partner for our auto-erotic sex-play.

Now, I live in the best of two worlds. I have a happy, successful marriage with a man I love. We have great sex, and I no longer feel frustrated about not being able to express my desire for my own manual pleasures. Because Ruth and I have become friends, each replacing the friend the other had in those formative teen years. We get together as often as we like, to watch each other masturbate. We both still derive explosive excitement from the activity. As long as our husbands don't know about it, nobody is threatened or hurt by it.

So please be sure and disguise my identity. I wouldn't want him to even suspect. But do be sure and tell my story to your readers. There may be others out there who feel frustrated because their mates disapprove of their simple pleasure. Maybe, like me, they can find someone to play with.

Procuress

Preston, thirty-six, is of medium height and slight build, with a receding hairline. His light blue eyes dart from side to side and blink nervously in time to a tic of some kind that causes his shoulders to rise in a series of involuntary shrugs as he speaks. Preston used to own a small neighborhood pharmacy, but now works for a large drugstore chain. He seems somewhat embarrassed as he tells us his story, almost as if he does not expect to be believed.

I'm no fool. I know what I look like. And I know that I don't appear to be the most masculine of men. Which is probably why I never thought this desire of mine would ever be anything more than a dream.

I've read your books and lots of other stuff about sex. So I realize that the thought of having two women at the same time is a typical male fantasy. Maybe the most popular male fantasy of all. Mine was a sort of variation on that theme.

Maybe it's because I look like a wimp. When I was in high school, the other guys used to make fun of me. Even my friends. If they were getting up a game of basketball or something, there would always be cracks about how Preston could be the timekeeper, or Preston can watch everybody's coats while they play. Nobody ever wanted me on their team, and that was all right with me, because I really didn't care for sports. I didn't like the way they kidded me. But they meant for it to be good-natured, so I just smiled through it.

While they played, I would sit on the sidelines and think about sex. In my imagination, I was the greatest cocksman that ever lived. Women would fall all over themselves fighting for me, and my only problem would be to decide which ones to fuck and in what order.

Actually, I did make out pretty well with the girls at school, even though I wasn't a football hero. For one thing, I didn't go after the gorgeous ones with big tits, like the other guys tended to do. To me, all girls were desirable, because of that magic spot they had between their legs. So at school socials, I'd dance with the ugly ones, the fat ones, the ones with bad complexions, the ones the other guys avoided like the plague. I'd talk sweet to them, and more often than not the evening would end in the back of my car with my hand up a girl's dress or down the front of her blouse. In the dark, it really didn't matter what they looked like. Meanwhile, the other guys were fumbling and bumbling and not getting any closer to real sex than a groping hand roaming awkwardly over the front of a girl's dress.

Well, girls talk to each other in the locker rooms just as much as boys do. The homely girls were so happy for my attention that they started bragging about the times they had with me. Word got around that I was a sexual artist. Then, even the attractive girls started showing an interest in me. In my junior year, I lost my virginity to the girl who was later elected homecoming queen. She lost hers to me at the same time. You might say we swapped cherries.

Unlike my pals, I never told any of the other guys about it. For one thing, I didn't want them to learn what I had learned, that romancing the ugly girls was a way of getting to the cute ones. More important, I wanted the girls to know that they were safe with me, that if they let me pet them or fuck them nobody would ever know about it.

So I'd sit there while the guys played ball, thinking about the girls I had been with and the ones I wanted to be with. I developed this fantasy in which I had a steady girlfriend who thought so much of my sexual ability that she started recommending me to all her friends, talking them into doing it with me, procuring for me. That would certainly make things easier, taking all the work out of seduction. But, even more, it would establish me as a sexual champion. I privately nursed that fantasy for years.

I came close to confessing it during a petting session with Nita, a girl I started dating while in college. Nita was one of those women that most other guys would ignore, because she was on the chubby side. But she had big, soft, floppy tits, which really turned me on. And the lack of male attention had made her horny as hell.

We were sitting in my car, which for me was like a motel on wheels, and her skirt was hiked up around her waist. I had my hand in her panties and was enjoying the wetness of her pussy. I kept telling her how excited she made me, as I ran my fingers up and down her pussy and toyed with the prominence of her clit. My words were turning her on as much as my hand was. She kissed me passionately, driving her tongue down my throat. Within moments, she was coming, groaning unintelligible sounds into my mouth as my fingers brought her to ecstasy.

When she was finished, she sighed deeply. "That was wonderful, Preston," she said. "Now I want to do something for you. Anything you'd like. Just tell me what you want."

My mind flashed to one of her friends, a curvaceous beauty who was the desire of every guy at the school. I was on the verge of saying, "If you really want to do something for me, get your friend to fuck me." But I realized how insulting this would sound, so I just said, "Would you suck my cock?"

She did, and it was great. The whole time, I was thinking about how hot it would be to have her and her friend taking turns licking me. Of course, I never let on. The secret of my success with women was that I always tried to make whoever I was with feel that I thought she was the sexiest female in the universe.

Nita was a really good sex partner. She was fat, but that didn't bother me at all. She was the most responsive woman

I'd ever known. It seemed like all I had to do was touch one of her nipples or dip my fingers in her pussy and she'd start humming like a machine, rocking her hips back and forth, getting all juicy and wet, and begging me to tell her what I wanted her to do for me.

She gave me lots of blowjobs in those days, because we both lived with our parents, and the only place we could find to be alone was in the back of my car. Once in a while, we'd fuck, with her sitting on my lap, right there on the seat. But as good as the sex was, it tended to be a bit uncomfortable.

Then one day when I went to pick her up, she asked if I'd like to go visit her married sister, Barb, who lived not far away. I wasn't crazy about the idea, but didn't exactly know how to say no, so I assented. She gave me directions and, as I drove, she explained that her sister had a spare bedroom and wouldn't mind if we used it for a few hours. The evening was beginning to sound a whole lot better.

When we got there, Barb greeted us at the door. She was a little taller than Nita, but had pretty much the same kind of figure—fleshy, with big, soft-looking boobs and a fat, rounded ass. She said her husband was out of town and offered us some wine. I sipped nervously, eager to get Nita into the bedroom. Barb watched me quietly and then said, "I know you'd like to be alone with Nita for a while, but maybe you'd both like a little dip in the hot tub first. It's right off the bedroom."

It sounded like a very sexy idea. We could fool around for a while in the hot water and get ready for some even hotter sex. "Why, thanks," I said. "But I don't have a bathing suit or anything."

"That's okay," she answered. "My husband and I love hot-tubbing in the nude. It's a lot more fun that way. In fact, if you don't mind, I'll join you." She led us through the spare bedroom to the tub, which was located in an enclosed porch, accessible through a sliding glass door.

At first, I was a little put off by the idea of her joining us. I couldn't very well fool around with Nita while her sister was right there watching. And it was going to be a little em-barrassing to be nude in front of my date's sister. But then I realized that from the way Barb had spoken, she probably intended to be nude, too. The prospect of seeing her naked overcame any negative feelings I had.

Sure enough, when we got to the tub, Barb unceremoni-ously removed all her clothes and stepped in. Her big pink nipples were hard, and I thought maybe she was excited by the idea of being nude in front of a stranger. Still, I hesitated until Nita had also undressed and climbed into the tub. Fi-nally, painfully conscious that both of them were watching me, I took off my clothes and prepared to join them. I was aware that my cock was hard and that the two women were looking at it. Nita giggled and said, "Looks like Preston's got some ideas in his mind." Barb joined her in laughter.

I eased into the water, grateful for the bubbles that almost hid my arousal. For a few minutes, we just sat there, the three of us soaking up the relaxation offered by the hot, churning water. I was embarrassed by the quiet, but couldn't think of anything to say. Trying to be unobtrusive, I glanced at the naked bodies of the two sisters, making a mental comparison as I imagined how it would be to have sex with each of them in turn.

At last Nita broke the silence. "Barb and I want to know something," she said in a voice that was barely audible over the sound of the hot tub pump.

"What's that?" I asked.

"Would you like to fuck Barb? Now, tell the truth."

I was stunned. How the hell was I supposed to answer a question like that? If I told the truth, that, yes, of course I'd like to fuck her, I was liable to piss them both off. But any other answer would be an obvious lie. Besides, she had asked for the truth.

I glanced at Nita, letting my gaze wander over the parts of her naked body that were exposed. Then I turned my sight to her sister, focusing on the softness of her tits, as they seemed to float on the water. When I looked into Barb's eyes,

217

she returned my gaze. I realized that the two women had talked about this in advance, prearranged it.

Still looking into Barb's eyes, I said, "Yes, I'd very much like to fuck Barb."

"Good," Nita said. "I'm going to watch." She got out of the tub and reached for my hand. I followed her back into the bedroom, with her sister right behind. "Now, Barb," Nita said. "You're going to see what I was talking about. Preston is going to give you the fucking of your life."

Still dripping wet, Barb lay down on her back on the bed and spread her legs wide to show me her pussy. The sight of it made my cock throb with desire. Knowing that Nita was watching made the whole thing seem surreal, like an erotic dream suddenly come to life. I got onto the bed between Barb's knees and leaned over to place my mouth against her sex.

Even though she had just come from the tub, there was a powerful musky fragrance wafting from her pussy, as though it was calling me and demanding my sexual attention. I started licking her, concentrating on the swollen bulb of her clit, until I felt her rising toward climax. Then I mounted her and drove my cock inside her pussy with one swift stroke. The moment I entered her, she started to come. I thrust in and out for a few moments and then I joined her, pouring my fluids into her to mix with her sweet secretions. It was over as quickly as it began.

I felt Nita stroking my bare ass, her fingers reaching down to caress my scrotum as my cock eased out of her sister's pussy. She took it in her hand, while it was thickly coated with the amalgam of my cum and Barb's all mingled together. Using the mixed juices as a lubricant, she massaged my cock until it was hard again. Then she lay on her back beside her sister and tugged me toward her.

I let her guide my cock to the opening of her pussy and entered her slowly, sliding all the way in and then stopping to let the full heat of her inner channel soak my organ. I tensed the muscles of my lower body, causing my cock to swell inside her, and then relaxed them as I drew back, bringing myself almost completely out of her until only my swollen cock head remained ensconced in her erotic warmth. Then I lowered myself and drove forward again.

I was conscious the whole time of Barb, lying next to us and watching our performance. She remained motionless as I fucked her sister, but murmured sounds of encouragement each time I plunged to the depths. We kept fucking and fucking until I felt I could hold out no longer. "I'm going to come," I whispered, speaking to both women at once.

"Yes," Nita responded. "Me too." It was the best orgasm I ever had, and I let Nita know it with the sounds I was making. I pressed my lips to hers and kissed her passionately, filled with a sense of love. She had given me her sister and now was giving me herself, two incredibly beautiful gifts. I couldn't believe my good fortune.

We made love for several hours after that, each of the women taking a turn, until I was totally exhausted. Before I collapsed, though, I managed to fuck Nita one last time, bringing cries of climax from her throat, even though I was too spent to come again myself. Afterwards, as I drifted off to sleep, I felt her kissing me tenderly, all over my body. When she got to my mouth, I could taste the scent of sex on her lips.

The following day, Nita told me that it had been the most exciting sex experience of her life. She explained that what she liked most about it was that after she had arranged for me to fuck another woman, I had made love to her with even greater gusto. She especially appreciated the fact that before falling asleep, I managed to fuck her one last time. She said it proved that I found her sexier than her sister, that it reaffirmed her belief in herself as a sexual being, that it made her feel superior to all the other women in the world.

One night a few weeks later, after we finished screwing in the backseat of my car, Nita said that she had a girlfriend she wanted me to meet. Someone she had told about me and who was interested in fucking me. Naturally, Nita planned to be there so that I could make love to her after fucking her friend. I was only too glad to oblige. It was similar to the experience we had with Barb, except that her friend was a real knockout. Still, I was careful to save my best stuff for Nita.

After that, Nita and I decided it was time for us to move in together. By pooling our resources, we managed to afford a small apartment. It wasn't much, but it seemed like a palace, because we got to sleep together every night and wake up together every morning. Best of all, a couple of times a month Nita would bring another woman over to spend the night with us.

My secret fantasy had come to life. The funny thing was that, no matter how many women Nita brought around for me to fuck, and no matter how good-looking they were or what great sex partners they turned out to be, I always found Nita sexier and more beautiful than anyone else. Before long, I was hopelessly in love with her.

We got married the day after I received my pharmacist's license and have lived happily ever after. She still brings other women into our bed and watches me fuck them. And she still takes delight in knowing that she turns me on more than any of the others. Lots of men spend their lives looking for paradise. I've found it.

Conclusion

$\mathscr{I}$f you're like most people, you probably have an unspoken desire of your own. Perhaps you have kept it secret because you consider it strange. Maybe you feel uncomfortable about it, fearful that it marks you as weird, or perverted, or deviant in some way.

We hope that this book has shown you that you are not alone in harboring private sexual desires. Lots of other people have feelings similar to your own. If the skeletons you have seen behind the closed doors that we opened for you are not exactly like your own, at least you have seen that anybody and everybody is likely to have one.

It would have been impossible for us to document all the secrets that have been described to us. There would not be enough paper on which to print them. Rest assured, however, that whatever your hidden erotic wishes may be, there probably are others who have similar ones.

You may have a good reason for keeping your desire unspoken. There are some erotic preferences that spouses really are not likely to accept or understand. On the other hand, it is evident from some of the stories we have retold that many people have a tendency to magnify the strangeness of their own fantasies or past experiences. We did not find them nearly as outlandish as they did themselves. You probably didn't either. Were they to disclose these secrets to their life partners, they might find willing participants in the activities about which they now feel so guilty.

We will not suggest that you divulge your own secret to your partner, only that you consider doing so. You will be the best judge of how your partner is likely to react. Remember the experiences of Craig and Olga in Chapter 11. Craig's wife discovered his secret voyeurism and joined him in it, leading them to a vastly improved sex life. However, when Olga's mate learned of her undisclosed exhibitionism, he walked out on her and ended their marriage.

These are vital considerations. It is also important to recognize and understand that there is nothing intrinsically wrong with keeping some sexual desires unspoken. We all have little fantasy worlds in which we can enjoy activities that might be prohibited to us in real life. It is not always necessary to do the things we imagine doing.

If you have an unspoken desire, you may want to keep it that way. You may want your spouse to go on believing that it is him or her alone who puts that special smile on your face when you are making love or preparing to do so. If, in spite of that decision, you still have a need to talk about it, feel free to tell us. We may repeat your story to the world, but we'll never let anyone know who you are.

Attention Readers

The authors have already begun gathering information for their next book. If you would like to participate by filling out a questionnaire, please get in touch with:

Iris and Steven Finz
P.O. Box 237
The Sea Ranch, CA 95497

Or É-mail us at:

huck@sexwriters.com

Or visit the authors' Web site for information and a questionnaire:

www.sexwriters.com